The
WATER
Prescription

For Health, Vitality, and Rejuvenation

CHRISTOPHER VASEY, N.D.

TRANSLATED BY JON E. GRAHAM

Healing Arts Press
Rochester, Vermont

Healing Arts Press
One Park Street
Rochester, Vermont 05767

Healing Arts Press is a division of Inner Traditions International

Copyright © 2002 by Éditions Jouvence
Translation © 2006 by Inner Traditions International

Originally published in French under the title *L'eau, source vitale de votre santé: Les méfaits de la déshydration* by Éditions Jouvence, S.A., Chemin du Guillon 20, Case 143, CH-1233 Genève-Bernex, Switzerland.

Note to the reader: This book is intended as an informational guide. The remedies, approaches, and techniques described herein are meant to supplement, and not to be a substitute for, professional medical care or treatment. They should not be used to treat a serious ailment without prior consultation with a qualified health care professional.

ISBN: 978-1-59477-095-1

Printed and bound in the United States of America

Text design and layout by Virginia L. Scott Bowman
This book was typeset in Sabon with Avenire as the display typeface

Contents

Introduction

It is said that water is the ideal drink for the human being, and that drinking water is good for one's health. The reasons why this would be the case, however, are rarely stated. As a consequence, water, as a drink, is often neglected as a factor in health.

This is especially unfortunate considering that water is so widely available and so low in cost.

Water plays a fundamental role in health. Drunk on a daily basis in sufficient quantity, it not only maintains the body in good working order but can also prevent and heal many disorders and health problems.

Who would imagine that fatigue, energy depletion, depression, eczema, rheumatism, high and low blood pressure, high cholesterol, gastric disorders, and premature aging could all be caused by a chronic lack of water in the body? Science has discovered that these problems—and a great many others—can be effectively prevented or treated by correct hydration.

Most people assume they are drinking enough fluids. Certainly they consume copious amounts of coffee, tea, and all sorts of soft drinks, but these beverages are far less effective in hydrating the body than plain water. Furthermore, in today's world, our bodies' need for water is much higher than it once was. Our food is too rich, too concentrated, and too salty, and the use of dehydrating substances such as alcohol and tobacco is very widespread. Stress, overheated and artificially ventilated homes, offices, and stores, air and water pollution—all contribute to our increased need for water.

As a consequence, large numbers of people do not realize that they are chronically dehydrated, much less that lack of water is the cause of many of their health problems. There is only one solution: drink a lot more water. But for people to make a permanent change in their habits, they need to know why water is so important. What exactly happens when water enters the body? What are the health conditions that can be traced to dehydration? How should we drink, and what water should we choose? These are just a few of the many questions answered in this book.

The final chapter presents ten simple remedies that show how drinking water as a therapeutic agent can have powerful curative effects.

1

Water and the Human Body

∽

Our image of how the body is constructed and our understanding of how it functions determine how we use the body and treat it in the event of illness.

Unfortunately, an old mechanistic vision of the body that has been disproved by current physiological research still survives —most often unconsciously—in the way we consider the body. This outdated concept can lead us to overlook a fundamental factor: the important role in health played by water.

The old concept, known as *solidism*, views the body as a machine made up of solid cogs (the organs) in which fluids circulate (blood, lymph). The body is constructed of a combination of "dry" and "hard" materials, with fluids or water constituting a negligible or very minor component whose role is limited to oiling the machinery and transporting different substances from one part of the body to another.

This way of looking at things so permeates our reasoning process that when an illness makes its presence known, we focus our attention on the solid parts of the body: the organs.

We give very little attention to the organic fluids from either a qualitative or, more important, a quantitative point of view.

Is there any justification for this lack of interest in the body's fluids? No, quite the contrary. In fact, what is the human body primarily constructed from, if not water?

THE BODY'S WATER CONTENT

Although the body is constructed of both liquid and solid materials, fluids are present in much greater quantity than solids. Physiology teaches us that water is actually the most important constituent of the body, accounting for 70 percent of the human body's composition.

A human body weighing around 150 pounds therefore consists of some 105 pounds of fluids (in the form of blood, lymph, and cellular fluids), representing a little over two thirds of the body's entire weight. The solid part of the body consists of only about 45 pounds. This is a far cry from a body built from "solid" materials with a little liquid thown in.

Furthermore, these figures are for the water content of an adult body. It is still higher during infancy, especially during the period of gestation. The body of a newborn is 80 percent water; that of a seven-month fetus, 85 percent; and that of a four-month fetus, 93 percent.

TABLE 1.1
THE BODY'S WATER CONTENT BASED ON AGE

Age	Water Content (%)
4-month fetus	93
7-month fetus	85
newborn	80
child	75
adult	70
elderly person	60

The fluids of the body are not all mixed together as if they were inside a large sack of skin. Rather, they are separated and allocated to different compartments throughout the body.

The fluid closest to the body's surface is blood. It is the first to receive substances taken in by the body from the outside, such as oxygen brought in by the respiratory tract and nutritive material passed through the mucous membranes of the digestive tract. The blood represents 5 percent of the body's weight, yet it circulates only within the arteries, veins, and capillaries of what is known as the vascular network.

Directly beneath the vascular network is another compartment containing extracellular fluid and lymph (figure 1.1).

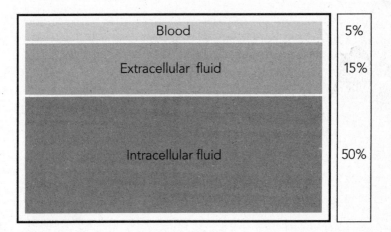

Figure 1.1. The three physical compartments or levels and their weight percentages in the body

As its name indicates, extracellular fluid is found outside the cells. It surrounds them like a bath, filling the small spaces or interstices that separate the cells from one another; it is also known as interstitial fluid. It forms the external environment of the cells, the great ocean in which they "float." This fluid receives oxygen (in fluid form) and nutritive substances carried by the bloodstream, and then it transports them to the cells, where this cargo is utilized. The extracellular fluid also receives the waste products and residues produced by the cells and transports them up to the higher compartment, the bloodstream, which in turn takes them to the excretory organs (liver, kidneys, etc.) so they can be filtered and eliminated (figure 1.2).

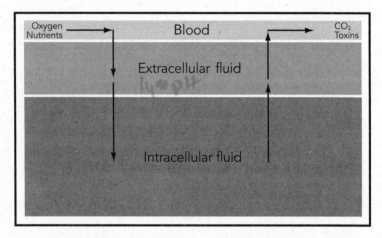

Figure 1.2. What the fluids transport

The lymph, which is located on the same level as the extracellular fluid, removes a portion of the toxins it has absorbed from the cells and carries it up to the bloodstream. The lymphatic vessels in which lymph circulates spill into the blood at the level of the subclavian arteries. From this point, the toxins are directed toward the excretory organs.

Together, extracellular fluid and lymph represent 15 percent of body weight, a weight three times greater than that of the blood. (To simplify this summary, from here on lymph and extracellular fluid are discussed as if they were a single fluid.)

The next compartment, the third and deepest, is that of the intracellular fluid. It is composed of all the liquids located within the cells.

Although the internal space of each individual cell is incredibly tiny, when all these spaces are put together, they nonetheless constitute a volume of considerable size. The intracellular fluid that fills them represents half the weight of the entire body.

The oxygen and nutrients carried here by the extracellular fluid penetrate into the intracellular fluid by traveling through the cellular membranes. Once inside the cell, they are used by the organs of the cell (the organelles) and by the cellular core (figure 1.3, see page 8).

The body—and hence the organs—consists of much more water than solid materials. The lungs and heart, for example, consist of 70.9 percent water; the muscles are 75 percent water; the liver is 75.3 percent; and the spleen is 77 percent. These percentages account for about 75 percent of the weight of the organs in question.

The brain is the organ with the highest fluid content, 83 percent. It has a proportionately high need for fluid to function properly. The brain alone receives 20 percent of the body's available blood supply, although it accounts for only 2 percent of total body weight.

So how is it that our bodies, with such a substantial proportion of liquid, seem so solid?

With the exception of a few organs or body parts (the skin, the nails), whose concentration of solid substances is quite high (78 percent for the skeleton), cells paradoxically acquire their solidity from the water that fills them. We can see the same phenomenon in an ordinary garden hose: soft and flexible when empty, it becomes rigid and firm when filled with water. The water that fills the cells exerts pressure on the cellular envelope, which gives the cells their shape and solidity.

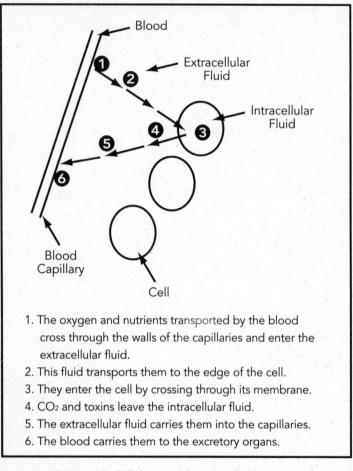

1. The oxygen and nutrients transported by the blood cross through the walls of the capillaries and enter the extracellular fluid.
2. This fluid transports them to the edge of the cell.
3. They enter the cell by crossing through its membrane.
4. CO_2 and toxins leave the intracellular fluid.
5. The extracellular fluid carries them into the capillaries.
6. The blood carries them to the excretory organs.

Figure 1.3. Cellular assimilation and elimination

There are such high quantities of water in the human body because the original environment from which all living species emerged was liquid. Water is therefore essential for life even to make an appearance.

WATER, THE ORIGINAL ENVIRONMENT
OF LIVING CREATURES

The first living creatures appeared in a marine environment. It was only thanks to a very slow process of evolution that certain animal species were able to leave that liquid environment to establish a partial foothold on solid ground, becoming amphibians. Later adaptive processes enabled some of these amphibians to leave the aquatic environment for good to make their homes permanently on solid ground.

Firm evidence that a marine environment was the original milieu from which all animal species have emerged was provided by the discovery that the composition of blood plasma (the fluid component of blood) and extracellular fluid of the different animal species is quite similar to the composition of seawater. This is true for not only the kinds of minerals present, but also their individual relative proportions.

Although the animal species living on land left the primordial ocean a long time ago, their dependence on water is still total. Cells still need to be bathed in a liquid to survive; and the regular, uninterrupted intake of water in sufficient quantity is absolutely essential to their function.

For the animals living in it, the sea represented not only their external environment but also an immense reservoir of water from which they could draw—in other words, drink—the entire time they were immersed in it. But the animal species that left the marine milieu to enter the dry, airy surroundings of terra firma no longer had an always-accessible reservoir of water from which they could serve themselves at any time.

For these creatures to survive, two things became indispensable: an internalization of the external fluid environment, and a very high-performance internal management system for the available water.

THE INTERNALIZATION
OF THE LIQUID ENVIRONMENT

Internalizing the liquid surroundings of the original marine milieu created the extracellular fluid in which the cells of land-based animal life forms now bathe. It forms a vast "inner ocean" in which the cells of our own bodies are located.

But internalizing the external water was not sufficient to ensure the survival of the organism. Henceforth functioning as an almost-closed circuit, the organism had to accomplish numerous tasks with a very limited quantity of water. Alexis Carrel, who won the Nobel Prize for Medicine in 1932, calculated that to irrigate properly a surface corresponding to the three-quarters of a square mile of cellular tissues in the human body would require some 200,000 liters of water! If the mere several dozen liters of liquid the human body requires to meet its needs are able to sustain life in all circumstances, it is because that liquid is not motionless but in constant movement.

Thanks to this movement, the cells of our tissues do not have to move to find food, as is partly the case for the single-celled organisms—amoebas, for example—in an aquatic milieu. Instead, food is brought to the cells by the fluids circulating throughout the body. Nor do the cells of the body have to find a way to distance themselves from the toxins they have recently released into their external environment, because the toxins are carried off by these same constantly moving liquids.

The different bodily fluids circulate at the speed most appropriate to them. Blood is the most rapid; it can make a circuit through the entire body in around a minute. The intra- and extracellular fluids move more slowly, but very rapid and very intense exchanges take place among the different levels. This is how the depths of the body—the cellular environment—can be rapidly affected by any substance entering the body. For example, several minutes is all it takes for the alcohol contained in a drink to enter the bloodstream, travel through the extracellular level and on into the cerebral cells, where its effects quickly become evident.

FLUID MANAGEMENT

The second essential for the survival of the organism is a management system that closely monitors the entrance and exit of all fluids, making sure that any deficit is rapidly compensated. Body fluids eliminated through urine, sweat, and so forth must be replaced by an intake of equal amounts of water.

The driving element of this management system is the sensation of thirst that pushes us to drink. It is triggered immediately when the body begins to dehydrate. If the water deficit becomes too great or endures for too long, it is the water we ingest that prevents us from withering away and dying. It takes only a few days of complete fluid deprivation—theoretically it is three days, but in practice it is closer to seven—for the body to cease functioning and die.

Our dependence on water is certainly not as great as our dependence on air; we can survive only a matter of minutes (approximately three to six minutes) without breathing. But air surrounds us; we are bathed in it, so it is always available, which is not the case for water.

Although thirst tells us when and how much we need to drink, we do not always absorb as much liquid as is necessary to enjoy the benefits of optimum health and vitality. This water deficit is not life-threatening, but it is enough to have negative consequences for our health. Like a plant that withers and droops from lack of water, a person suffering from partial dehydration loses strength and energy and becomes ill. Unfortunately, the cause of the illness often goes unrecognized.

Qualitatively and quantitatively, the importance of water is at the core of the approach called *humorism* (from the old meaning of the word *humor,* which was used to refer to the various body fluids). Contrary to solidism, which considers the body an aggregate of solid and dry organs and views healing as actions directed at the organs, humorism views the body as a collection of fluids in which the cells are bathed and on which they are deeply dependent. Anything affecting the quality or the quantity of these fluids (intra- and extra-cellular fluids, lymph, and blood) creates health problems whose seriousness is in proportion to the degree of variance from the optimum state. The therapeutic methods advocated by humorism aim to maintain and restore the ideal condition of the fluids. Humorism is the basis of all medical systems that deal with the internal cellular environment (naturopathy, homeopathy, and so on).

To the proponents of humorism, water is not merely an accessory element useful for filling empty spaces (its structural role) and carrying nutrients (its role as a transporter); it plays a fundamental role in the very functioning of the body. Water is not just *used* by the solid parts but has a direct effect on these parts by virtue of its presence, motion, and properties.

The functions performed by water are many:

Energetic. By entering and exiting the cells, water produces hydroelectric energy that is stored in the form of adenosine triphosphate, or ATP.

Hydrolytic. Water triggers chemical reactions by decomposing the substances suspended in it.

Activating/inhibiting. The thicker body fluids become, the more slowly biological reactions take place, which means that a sufficient intake of liquid enables the body's organic "motor" to resume its normal operating speed.

Eliminatory. The purification of the blood by the kidneys occurs because of the pressure applied to the renal filter by the liquid carried there by the renal artery.

Thermoregulatory. When water evaporates on the skin, it cools the body.

Circulatory. The quantity of water in the body regulates blood pressure and the movement of the blood.

Osmotic. The numerous exchanges that take place between the inside and outside of the cells occur as a result of the different pressures applied by the fluids located in various parts of the cellular membranes.

Furthermore, it turns out that the heart is better described not as a pump that makes fluids circulate throughout the body but as an exchanger that is set in motion and kept working by the fluids themselves (circulatory function). Corroboration of the experiments performed in this area by Professor Leon Manteuffel-Szoege* is provided by the fact that, in the fetus, the circulatory system is formed and begins to function before the heart.

Therefore not only is water present in the body's structure in much greater quantity than is commonly believed, but it also plays a fundamental role in the body's physical functioning.

Having examined some of the little-known roles played by water in the body, we now turn to the ways water enters the body, what happens once it has entered, and how it exits the body.

---

*"Réflexions sur la nature des functions mécaniques du coeur" [Thoughts on the Heart's Mechanical Functions]

2

The Cycle of Water in the Body

〜

The body is the transit zone for an uninterrupted flow of water. This journey consists of three stages: the intake of water, its absorption by the cells and tissues, and its elimination.

WATER INTAKE

The water the body requires to meet its needs enters it by three paths of unequal importance: the mouth, the lungs (in the form of steam), and the skin.

Mouth

The principal path taken by water to enter the body is through the mouth. Every day, we ingest around 2.5 liters of liquid by mouth. This liquid can be in a free form or bound with other substances.

Free form is the liquid we ingest by itself, or combined with substances that give it a specific color, flavor, and aroma: ground coffee to make a stimulating beverage, leaves from medicinal plants to make infusions, and sugar and natural or artificial flavors to make soft drinks.

Water bound with other substances refers to water that is naturally part of the tissues of the solid foods we eat, such as the juice contained in the pulp of fruits and vegetables. As water is essential for all forms of life, all our foods—whether they are of plant or animal origin—are also formed with water. Some, however, are richer in water than others. Just what is the water content of different kinds of food?

The foods that have the highest water content are vegetables. The absolute record is held by cucumbers, which have a water content of 95.6 percent. Salad greens run a close second with a water content reaching 94.4 percent, and escarole, 94 percent exactly. Root vegetables have a slightly lower content: 88.6 percent for carrots, 88 percent for celery, and 86.8 percent for beets. Of course, the way vegetables are prepared for eating also plays a role in their water content. Although potatoes are composed of 77.4 percent water and maintain close to this level when boiled or steamed (76 percent), their water content drops drastically when they are turned into fries (20 percent) and chips (3 percent).

Fruits are almost as juicy as vegetables. The fruits richest in water are watermelons and other members of the melon family (92 percent). The most commonly eaten fruits, such as apples and pears, have a water content of about 84 percent. Dried fruits, as their name suggests, contain much less liquid: raisins and dried apricots are 24 percent water, while dates are 20 percent. Oleaginous (oily) fruits like nuts have even less water content: almonds have 4.7 percent and hazelnuts, merely 3 percent.

The water content of animal foods is around 70 percent, similar to that of the human body. Fish have a slightly higher content (between 65 and 82 percent). Eggs are again almost the same as the human body (74 percent), whereas meats are slightly lower (from 56 to 70 percent). Chicken has 70 percent; veal, 69 percent; lamb, 62 percent; beef, 61 percent; and pork, 56 percent. Cold cuts and prepared meats have a much lower liquid content, ranging from 15 to 50 percent: liver pâté has 37 percent; salami, 28 percent.

Dairy products rich in liquid include yogurt (86 percent) and soft white cheese (e.g., cottage cheese, mozzarella, low-fat cream cheese, and farmer cheese, at up to 79 percent). These are high percentages when you realize that the cow's milk from which these products are manufactured has a water content of 87 percent. Soft cheeses such as goat cheeses and Camembert contain 53 percent water, but harder cheeses (Swiss cheese, Jarlsberg, Gruyère, Emmenthal) have only 34 percent.

Cereal grains (wheat, rice, rye, and so on) all have a water content bordering on 12 percent when dry. Once they have been boiled and have absorbed water, this percentage rises sharply to around 71 percent. The same goes for dried pasta and noodles. Uncooked they contain 9 percent water; when cooked their fluid content reaches 61 percent. Because cereal flakes are merely crushed grain, their water content is virtually identical to that of raw grain. In contrast, the water content of bread varies from 34 to 37 percent, while that of crackers and toast is closer to 7 and 8 percent.

Legumes such as lentils, chickpeas, white beans, and soybeans have a water content similar to that of cereal grains, around 11 percent.

Refined sugar contains no water. Candies have about 4.5 percent and chocolate 1 percent.

As water content is only one of the numerous characteristics of food, it cannot be used on its own as a criterion for setting up a diet plan. Certain foods are essential for maintaining a balanced diet despite their very low water content (cereal grains, for example), whereas others that have an extremely high water content, such as watermelon, are of negligible value nutritionally.

A person's water intake may be high or low depending on the foods in his or her basic diet. It is elevated if the person eats lots of fruits and vegetables, but reduced if these foods represent only a small portion of the daily diet. For some people, the water in fruits and vegetables fulfills up to two-thirds of their daily needs, with the final third supplied by drinks. For others, these proportions are reversed; the solid-food portion of their diet is much drier because of its lack of fruits and vegetables, so two-thirds of their daily water needs must be covered by drinks.

TABLE 2.1. THE WATER CONTENT OF FOOD (%)

VEGETABLES	
Cucumbers	95.6
Salad greens	94
Green peppers	90.4
Broccoli	90
Green and red cabbage	90
Turnips	89
Carrots	88.6
Celery	88
Beets	86.8
Onions	85
Potatoes	77.4
Peas	75
Garlic	65
FRUITS	
Tomatoes	97
Watermelon, melons	92
Papaya	91
Grapefruit	90

FRUITS (CONTINUED)	
Cranberries	89
Peaches	89
Oranges	87
Apricots (raw)	87
Blackberries	85
Apples, pears	84
Mangoes	84
Blueberries	80
Raisins	24
Almonds	4.7
Hazelnuts	3
MEATS	
Chicken	70
Veal	69
Lamb	62
Beef	61
Pork	65
Salami	28
FISH	
Cod	82
Pollack	80
Trout	77.6
Mackerel	68.1
Salmon	65.5
EGGS	
Hen's eggs	74
DAIRY PRODUCTS	
Cow's milk	87
Yogurt	86
Soft white cheese	79
(e.g., fromage blanc,	
cottage cheese, mozzarella,	

DAIRY PRODUCTS (CONTINUED)

low-fat cream cheese, farmer cheese)	
Crème fraîche, sour cream	62
Camembert	53
Roquefort	40
Cheddar	38
Cantal	37
Swiss, Gruyère	34
Parmesan	31
Butter	17.4

CEREAL GRAINS

Wheat	12.6
Rice (uncooked)	12
Rice (cooked)	71
Barley	11.1
Oats	11
Pasta (uncooked)	9
Pasta (cooked)	61

BAKED GOODS

Crackers	7–8
Bread	34–37

LEGUMES

White beans	16.7
Lentils	11.6
Chickpeas	10.6
Soybeans	7.5

CONDIMENTS AND MISCELLANEOUS FOODS

Mayonnaise	40
Jelly	30
Honey	20
Candy	4.5
Sugar (refined)	0

Lungs

The second way water can enter the body is via the respiratory tract. Water suspended in the air in the form of invisible vapor makes contact with the mucous membranes when the air is inhaled. Absorption of the humidity of the air takes place around the level of the alveoli, although not much water is taken in in this manner. The absorption process occurs passively and is not highly developed in human beings. Some insects, in contrast, fill an appreciable portion of their water requirements by drawing the water held by the air through their respiratory tracts, and they are able to do this even when the relative humidity of the air is quite low.

Skin

The skin also provides a means for water to enter the body. As with the respiratory tract, the amount of water absorbed by the body through the skin is fairly small. This is a protective mechanism, because if the skin could absorb generous amounts of the water with which it came in contact, the body would expand dangerously in size every time it was immersed in water.

There are some therapies that take advantage of the skin's capacity to absorb water. For example, it is used as a complementary means of rehydrating individuals who are suffering from sunstroke and have lost large quantities of bodily fluid and salt through sweat. Such people are gradually rehydrated by being given slightly salted water to drink, but also by being wrapped in cloths that have been soaked in water to restore fluid through the skin, as well as to prevent any additional dehydration.

The skin and lungs are not the major means of intake to cover the body's daily water requirements. The primary path is the digestive tract.

In addition to the three ways listed above, the body has one other source for the water it needs: metabolic fluid.

Metabolic Fluid

Metabolic fluid does not come from outside the body but from within. The body itself produces it, not from the water contained in foods, but by using the solid components of the foods ingested.

Metabolic fluid is produced by the transformation of fats and carbohydrates into energy. The different chemical transformations these substances undergo lead to the production of usable energy (the energy used by the muscles), and the creation of nonusable energies: the metabolic wastes and residues (or toxins) that need to be expelled from the body. This includes carbon dioxide (CO_2) that is breathed out by the lungs and water (H_2O). The latter is generally said to be eliminated by the lungs in the form of a vapor, or by way of the urinary tract. It is not eliminated directly by these organs, however, as it is produced in the cells and has to travel through the body before reaching the excretory organs. As the water being eliminated makes its way through the body, it contributes to the hydration of the physical tissue.

A human being produces around 300 grams, or 0.66 pound, of metabolic fluid per day. This nonnegligible contribution is not one of the human body's main priorities. Some animal species are much more dependent on this source of liquid than we are; in some cases it is their main source of liquid. The most extreme case is that of the jerboa, a desert rodent that seems capable of going without water entirely. The water its body needs is furnished primarily by its metabolic fluids, and to a small extent the water that is bound to the solid components of the food it eats: grains that have about a 10 percent water content. Of course, the small intake of liquid is compensated for by measures that limit its loss. The jerboa sweats less than other animals, it urinates much less, and its stools are quite dry. Furthermore, it spends its days in underground tunnels protected from the sun and heat, only venturing out at night.

The ability to produce metabolic fluid is one of the factors in the proverbial resistance of camels to heat and lack of water. The camel's hump does not contain water, as is sometimes thought, but fat. This fat forms an energy reserve that is oxidized when necessary to produce metabolic water.

TABLE 2.2. WATER INTAKE (AVERAGE, IN LITERS)

Drinks	1.2
Water from foods	1.0
Metabolic fluid	0.3
Total	2.5

ABSORPTION OF WATER

For humans and most animals, water is ingested primarily through the digestive tract. To reach the depths of the tissue, water must first leave this canal. It does this primarily via a process called osmosis, which occurs when water has to cross through a membrane or pass from one physical compartment of the body to another. Given the importance of osmosis, a detailed description follows.

Osmosis

Osmosis occurs when two liquids of different density are separated by a permeable tissue. The water's movement (the osmotic transfer) goes from the least concentrated environment—the one with less solid substance in suspension—to the more highly concentrated, until the density of both liquids has become equal. The transfer takes place because the more concentrated fluid exerts pressure on the fluid that is less concentrated. Because the membrane that separates the more dilute from the more concentrated fluid is permeable, the water in the dilute fluid moves toward the concentrated fluid and reduces its concentration. At the same time, the remaining dilute fluid becomes denser because it has transferred some of its water to the concentrated fluid, and balance is thus achieved between the two (figure 2.1, see page 24).

The amount of fluid transferred from one side of the membrane to the other is proportionate to the strength of the osmotic pressure, meaning the difference in concentration between the fluid on one side and the fluid on the other. If the fluids on both sides of the membrane are in balance and the pressure is equal, the net flow is zero.

Some membranes have a so-called selective permeability, which means that, in addition to water, they allow the passage of very specific solid substances such as minerals, glucose, and so on. The transfer of the solid substances usually goes in the opposite direction from the transfer of fluid, thus allowing an easier and quicker balancing of the two fluids. The more concentrated environment reduces its concentration both by the intake of water and by the outflow of solid substances.

The membranes of cells are selective. They allow potassium to enter but not sodium or chloride. These last two elements, which when combined produce sodium chloride or regular table salt, are consequently found on the cells' exterior.

This does not mean that sodium never enters the cells, however. Along with the passive phenomenon of osmosis, there is another, active method that enables the cells to absorb substances that the normal permeability of their walls would prevent. This absorption is achieved through the help of pumps, the best known of which is the sodium pump. These pumps

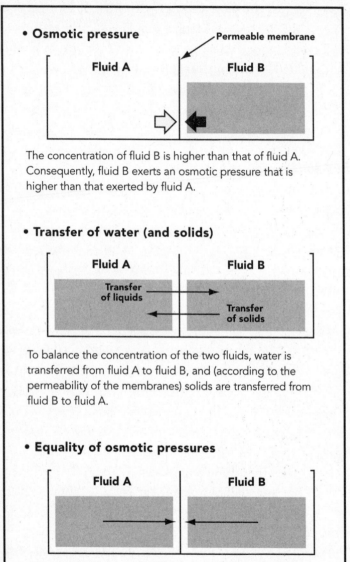

• Osmotic pressure

Fluid A **Fluid B** Permeable membrane

The concentration of fluid B is higher than that of fluid A. Consequently, fluid B exerts an osmotic pressure that is higher than that exerted by fluid A.

• Transfer of water (and solids)

Fluid A **Fluid B**

Transfer of liquids

Transfer of solids

To balance the concentration of the two fluids, water is transferred from fluid A to fluid B, and (according to the permeability of the membranes) solids are transferred from fluid B to fluid A.

• Equality of osmotic pressures

Fluid A **Fluid B**

The transfers have created a balance in the concentration of the two fluids. Their osmotic pressures are equal, and the osmotic exchanges have come to a halt for the time being.

Figure 2.1. Osmotic exchanges

allow the cells, based on their needs, to draw in substances on the other side of their membrane that are useful to them.

These osmotic exchanges that take place at the level of all the membranes and mucous areas of the body allow the tissues to absorb water and permit the ceaseless exchange and movement of fluids from one "story" or layer of the body to the next.

Exchange between Intestines and Blood

To make its way into the tissues, the water in the digestive tract must first cross through its walls so it can enter the bloodstream. As absorption is done through osmosis, it is naturally very weak in the mouth. The blood capillaries underneath the tongue allow some absorption of water, but water is not in contact with them long enough for significant absorption to take place.

In the stomach, absorption is also quite weak, because the primary function of this organ is digestion and not incorporation. Water travels rapidly through the stomach to reach the intestines, whose main function is incorporation. When the intestines are already holding a sufficient volume of water, the stomach temporarily holds onto the excess water and only releases it when the intestinal water content goes down (the regulating function of water's passage through the stomach).

The mucous membrane lining the small intestine is carpeted with blood capillaries. The membrane that separates the inside of the intestine from the capillaries is only a single layer of cells thick, no more than 0.0030 millimeter. Osmotic exchanges take place easily here, especially since ingested food and drink remain in contact with the intestinal mucus for a long time.

Water is therefore primarily absorbed at the level of the small intestine, as is also the case with nutritive substances. In fact, 90 percent of the water that is drunk or bound with foods enters the bloodstream from the small intestine, and more specifically the upper half of the small intestine.

When someone drinks without eating, the fluid the small intestine receives has a lower concentration of substances than the blood. The blood contains the numerous substances it transports (glucose, minerals, and so forth) and its own components (red corpuscles, platelets, and others). The solid substances contained in blood represent 10 percent of its weight, compared to those in water at 1 percent. The osmotic pressure is thus stronger from the blood side, which produces a transfer of water from the intestines into the bloodstream. This transfer takes place quite rapidly, as we notice if we observe how quickly the sensation of thirst is satisfied after drinking something. Several minutes are enough for water to enter the bloodstream and allow the body to give us the signal that our thirst has been quenched. The time necessary for an overdose of fluid to enter the bloodstream, which increases its volume too much and triggers corrective excretion from the area of the kidneys, is almost as short.

This situation does not change fundamentally when drinks are consumed along with food. The water absorption occurs with the same ease, but a little more slowly. Obviously the mixture of solid foods and liquids creates a fluid whose density is higher than straight water. This density is not very high, however, as it is necessary for the alimentary bolus (the mass of chewed food) to be fairly fluid in order to move forward as it flows toward the bottom of the digestive tract. The density of the alimentary bolus is also mitigated partially by the abundant secretion of digestive juices (as much as 7 liters a day), and partially by the water contained in the food. The concentration of the alimentary bolus is reduced enough so that its density is less than that of blood. This comes about quite easily; throughout the digestive process, nutritive substances leave

Chew food well

the intestinal environment (reducing the concentration of the alimentary bolus) and enter the blood, temporarily increasing its density. The osmotic pressure exerted by the blood therefore remains higher, and the passage of water from the intestine into the blood takes place smoothly. The small intestine's ability to absorb water is almost limitless. In practice, we can drink as much water as we want, and the water is always assimilated. Never—except in the case of a huge overdose of water, or if the intestines are extremely sensitive—does it flow out of the body directly by way of the intestines.

Despite the small intestine's strong absorption capacity, the alimentary bolus that leaves it to move into the large intestine still contains about a liter of water. The mucous layer of the colon absorbs this water, but only partially. The presence of water is essential to ensure the elimination of stools. Elimination takes place when the water content of the stools has reached a very precise percentage of their entire weight. Several percentages less, and they become too hard and cause constipation; several percentages higher, and they become too liquid and cause diarrhea.

The passage of water into the bloodstream from the intestine, along with the passage that takes place later of blood to the lower area of the body, does not occur at the level of the arteries and veins but at the capillaries. Given the importance of the capillary vessels to the topic of this book, a digression for a brief description of their characteristics is in order.

Capillaries

Capillaries are extremely thin and fragile blood vessels. They are often compared to hairs (hence their name, from the Latin word for hair, *capillaris*). In reality, they are much thinner than hairs: their diameter is somewhere between 5 and 30 microns (a micron is one thousandth of a millimeter, or 0.00004 inch). They are so small that red blood corpuscles can only travel through them in single file. The progress of the corpuscles is immediately interrupted if the capillaries contract.

Capillaries are so numerous because it is their role to irrigate the depths of the tissues. They do so by dividing up and spreading out in branches—like a tree—to irrigate every part of the body. If the arteries and veins could be compared to the large highways that cross a country, the capillaries would be the hundreds of thousands of small secondary roads and private drives that serve every house (or cell).

The capillary walls are permeable and allow the passage of water and nutritive substances, as well as toxins released by the cells. Although the capillaries are small, the entire capillary network, if stretched out in a single line, would equal 25,000 miles (40,000 kilometers). If all the arteries, veins, and capillaries in the human body were placed end to end, the total length would equal more than 60,000 miles (100,000 km)—they could stretch around the Earth nearly two and a half times, and their exchange surface would measure an acre and a half (6,300 square meters; the equivalent of a surface more than a mile in length and more than a yard in width, or 6 kilometers long and 1.05 meters wide). This is the gigantic surface from which everything that enters the body from outside (by way of the digestive tract, the lungs, and so forth) reaches the inner tissues, and from which everything released by the tissues, such as toxins, is carried out of the body.

The quantity of blood held by the body is not enough to completely fill the arteries and veins and the whole of the capillary network simultaneously. This is why the capillaries of the areas of the body that are at rest—a muscle, for example—contract to expel the blood they contain and make it available to the capillaries of the active organs or other parts of the body being used. This explains, for example, the experience of sleepiness after a meal, when the capillaries of the digestive tract are gorging on blood to the detriment of the capillaries of the brain.

The vasoconstricting (narrowing) and vasodilating (expanding) abilities of the capillaries also permit them to handle variations of fluid intake. The capillaries dilate when a large amount of water enters the blood and thus increases its volume; they contract when the opposite situation prevails.

Exchange between Blood and Extracellular Fluid

More than 95 percent of the water that enters the body by means of the digestive tract can be found in the blood. The increase in the volume of this water in proportion with what we drink, however, is limited; otherwise the blood vessels would expand to the point of bursting from the increased pressure of the water. But osmotic exchanges rapidly reduce blood volume (in tandem with the subtraction of liquid from the blood performed by the kidneys, a process to be examined later).

The water that enters the bloodstream from the digestive tract dilutes the blood and reduces its osmotic pressure on the walls of the blood vessels (the osmotic pressure of a fluid is not caused by its volume but by its concentration). On the other side of the walls of the vessels is the extracellular fluid, whose concentration of solid substances is quite close to that of blood. This similarity enables the body, with very slight changes in the concentration of the blood or extracellular fluid, to direct the osmotic transfers in one direction or the other as needed. These transfers move from the blood to the extracellular fluid for assimilation of nutrients, and from the extracellular fluid to the blood for elimination of toxins.

When the blood becomes less concentrated because of the intake of liquid, the extracellular fluid acquires greater density, which triggers the osmotic transfer of water from the blood into the extracellular fluid. As this process takes place continually, the excess water in the blood leaves it almost as soon as it arrives.

The water that enters the interstitial compartment is used to renew the extracellular fluid into which the cells have deposited their wastes. It also permits the interstitial environment to give up water to the cells without running the risk of drying out. The cells have an acute need for water, and their sole source is the fluid from the interstitial environment. The cells are, in fact, irrigated by the blood only indirectly (see figure 1.3, page 8).

Normally, thanks to control mechanisms, the volume of extracellular fluid remains stable. It can vary, however. A deficit of liquid at this level leads to dehydration of the tissues and thereby to a number of disorders, which are discussed later in the book. Excess liquid in the interstitial region is the prime cause of edemas, or abnormal accumulations of fluid in the tissues. Edemas arise not from an increase in cell volume but from an increase in volume of certain portions of the interstitial compartment. Such swellings can occur in the legs (most often around the ankles), the hands (making it difficult to remove rings), or the eyelids. This disorder is most often the result of an excess of salt. Some salt is normal, because one of the properties of salt is the retention of water—11 grams of water to 1 gram of salt—but salt in excess is harmful.

Exchange between Extracellular Fluid and Cells

The cells are the final destination of the water that enters the body. They are where the numerous biochemical transformations take place that are necessary to ensure the body's proper functioning. Seventy percent of the water contained in the body is found in the cells.

The water in the extracellular fluid is able to enter the cells either by means of osmosis or with the help of tiny special pumps that are scattered over the surface of the cell. These pumps allow better monitoring and more finely tuned management of the liquid intake than would be possible with osmotic exchanges alone.

Inside each cell, water serves as the basic building block for the intracellular fluid needed to fill each cell. It also serves to renew this liquid, to transport substances from one part of the cell to another, and to play many other roles in the life of the cell.

For the cells to perform their functions successfully, they must contain an optimum amount of water. Any quantitative variation in this content is a potential cause of various disturbances and illnesses, so the body responds immediately to any and all changes in its hydric volume. A liquid deficiency mobilizes the cells to draw water from the extracellular fluid. Conversely, any excess of water is rapidly corrected by its expulsion from the cells back into the extracellular fluid.

Constant exchanges in both directions are taking place through the cellular membrane that separates the extracellular and intracellular areas. These exchanges are vigorous and constitute a rapid, continual renewal of the liquids that make up the body.

Return Path

As it passes through the gears of the cellular engine, water becomes "worn out" and must be removed from the cell so that the body can eliminate it. This worn-out water is not only devitalized, containing fewer vitamins and minerals, but it is also laden with the toxins produced by the cell.

To leave the body, water ascends back into the extracellular fluid, then makes its way into the blood so the blood can carry it to the excretory organs responsible for the elimination of water and wastes. With this, the entire cycle of water in the body has run its course.

Given the high sensitivity of the cells to the qualities and defects of their environment, a constant replenishment of organic fluids must take place. And although the body essentially replaces all the solid parts of which it is made in the space of seven years, its renewal of liquids takes only two to three weeks.

ELIMINATION OF WATER

Water is eliminated from the body by four different routes.

Kidneys

The kidneys are the principal excretory organ for the elimination of water. Every day we eliminate 1 to 1.5 liters of water in the form of urine. When it passes through the renal glomeruli (the small filters that make up the kidneys), a portion of the water contained in the blood is removed along with various solid wastes (worn-out minerals, uric acids, urea, and so forth). Together, this water and these solid substances compose the urine. Urine is 95 percent water and 5 percent solids.

There are about one million glomeruli in each kidney. Filtering occurs primarily as a result of the different pressures on either side of the glomerular membrane. Because the pressure is stronger on the blood side, the water is stripped of some of its constituent parts in the same way that pressure applied to a mesh bag holding fruit puree squeezes jelly out through the mesh. The role of pressure in the filtration process explains why the production of urine and the need to urinate increases when blood pressure rises (such as with stage fright, after drinking coffee, or when swimming in very cold water); this pressure is weaker in people who have low blood pressure.

Among the different animal species, the quantity of water eliminated by the kidneys depends very much on how proteins are metabolized. Proteins can provide two kinds of waste products: urea and uric acid.

Urea requires a great deal of water not only to be transported, but also for sufficient dilution of the urine so it does not irritate the mucous membranes of the urinary system. This dilution is reached in the human being when the volume of urine eliminated in one day is approximately 1.5 liters. Most urea comes from the metabolism of proteins. The volume of urea that proteins generate is relatively large compared to that generated by other nutritive elements.

Certain animals, however—such as birds and reptiles—urinate very little, and their urine is thick. With these creatures, the metabolism of proteins leads essentially to the formation of uric acid, a substance that is not soluble in water and retains a solid consistency. This is why birds, for example, do not urinate liquid like most animals but excrete a thick and viscous substance.

In addition to their purifying effect on the blood, the kidneys—among other organs—monitor the body's liquid content. When water intake is insufficient and the tissues are lacking fluid, the kidneys excrete wastes using smaller volumes of water. Conversely, if the body is currently taking in too much water, the kidneys eliminate more water than normally.

Skin

Water leaves the body through the skin in the form of sweat. Sweat is composed of 99 percent water and 1 percent solid substances. The latter are worn-out minerals (sodium, phosphorus, and so forth) or organic wastes (urea, uric acid, and others). Sweat eliminates the same wastes as the kidneys, but in a less concentrated form (recall that urine contains

5 percent solid wastes, compared to 1 percent in sweat).

Sweat is produced and eliminated by the sudoriferous glands; we have between 70 and 120 of these for every square centimeter of skin. The filtering process performed by these glands is identical to that performed by the renal glomeruli: the difference in the pressure on either side of the filter causes the passage of a portion of the water and wastes held by the blood into the sudoriferous glands. The sweat formed in this way then makes its way to the surface of the skin by means of very slender ducts.

Sweat permits the elimination of wastes and the water whose healthful properties have been used up by the body, but it also regulates the body temperature when it has risen too steeply due to ambient heat, physical exertion, or fever. The evaporation of the water on the surface of the skin removes heat from the body and cools it down. Perspiration and the resulting water loss are therefore greater the more body temperature has increased.

Perspiration occurs in two degrees of volume. In the lower-volume degree, moisture is constantly being excreted from the body through the skin but in extremely fine droplets that are invisible to the naked eye and evaporate the moment they reach the skin. The higher-volume degree of sweating, however, takes place only episodically. Its chief characteristic is the visibly abundant release of sweat.

Every minute, approximately 0.03 gram of sweat is produced by all the sudoriferous glands of the body, which amounts to some 540 grams (1.2 pounds) every twenty-four hours. This figure represents the sweat produced when the body is at rest and which leaves the body in the form of perspiration. During intense physical activity, this figure can climb as high as 1 liter or more per hour. During times of high heat, the removal of liquid from the blood to form sweat increases further. In a sauna, a person excretes 40 grams of sweat a minute, or 1,200 grams (2.6 pounds) in a half-hour. Patients with high fevers may eliminate as much as 5 to 6 liters of sweat a day. But this is possible only if the water lost is being constantly replaced by ingestion. The ingested water is transferred from the intestinal region to the bloodstream, from where it goes into the sudoriferous glands. If the amount of water drunk is insufficient to make up for the losses, the liquid is no longer taken from the intestine, but from the extracellular fluid. If this is still not enough, it begins to be drawn from even deeper fluid reserves, those in the cells. When these withdrawals are of substantial size or are repeated over an extended period, a state of dehydration becomes established. The production of sweat diminishes, and the sweat the body releases is more concentrated. It is imperative that water be drunk to reestablish the body's hydric balance.

The skin of some animals, such as dogs, does not allow them to perspire sufficiently to lower their body temperature after intense physical effort. For these animals, the evaporation process takes place in the lungs. By lolling their tongues and panting, they are creating via the respiratory tract an evaporation process similar to what takes place in the human being via the skin.

Lungs

When we exhale, a certain amount of liquid leaves the body in the form of vapor. This passive elimination of water releases between 300 and 500 grams (or 0.66 and 1.1 pounds) a day. The volume increases during intense physical activity (2 to 5 milliliters a minute, as opposed to 0.25 a minute when the body is at rest) and also during dry, hot weather, because a certain level of humidity needs to be maintained in the lungs so that the respiratory mucous membranes do not dry out. When the membranes become dry, they become more fragile and inflexible, which can lead to problems such as coughing.

Intestines

The intestines eliminate the smallest amount of water from the body. Although the 150 grams (0.33 pound) of stool that the human being eliminates daily can have a solid appearance, its liquid content can be as high as 120 grams (0.26 pound). This liquid is necessary to facilitate evacuation. In some intestinal disorders, the presence of water and its elimination reach abnormally high levels (several liters). The stools then become liquid, and what we call diarrhea occurs.

An excess of water in the stools can have one of two explanations.

In noncontagious diarrhea, an agitated nervous system or foods that irritate the intestinal mucous membrane (hard-to-digest food, or food that is spoiled or fermented) cause this membrane to secrete excessively. These are protective secretions to dilute the stools so that they are less harmful. When this process is used regularly by the body, it loses a great quantity of water and this tends to lead to dehydration.

In infectious diarrhea, viruses or bacteria destroy the cells of the intestinal wall, which prevents the intestines from absorbing the liquid from drinks, foods, and digestive juices. This excessive quantity of water greatly dilutes the stools and gives them a liquid consistency. The water is no longer making its way into the bloodstream or the cells, and thus there is a high risk of dehydration since the digestive tract is the principal entryway into the body for the water it ingests.

⤳

This look at the elimination of liquids brings us to the end of the water cycle in the body. The passage of water through every level (digestive, blood, extracellular, intracellular, then the same path in the opposite direction as water leaves the body) is only one aspect of the water cycle. Within this large cycle, water travels through smaller cycles, including one in relation to the digestive tract and another involving the kidneys. These are discussed next to demonstrate how the body, which functions partially as a closed circuit, is dependent on the constant circulation of fluids to remain alive.

TABLE 2.3. LIQUID LOSSES (AVERAGE, IN LITERS)

Urine	1.5
Sweat	0.5
Through the lungs	0.4
Through the intestines	0.1
Total	2.5

Digestive Tract

To produce their secretions, the digestive glands obtain the water they need from the blood. The amount of this water withdrawal is not negligible; every day the human digestive tract secretes around 7 liters of digestive juices: 1 liter of saliva, 1.5 liters of gastric juice, 0.75 liter of bile, 0.75 liter of pancreatic juices, and 3 liters of intestinal juices.

Although these secretions are created at the expense of the water in the blood, the blood volume is not reduced. The blood rebuilds itself from the liquid provided by drinks and foods, as well as what is provided by the digestive tract itself. Digestive juices used to break down and liquefy foods are not eliminated with the stools at the end of the digestive process but are in large part reabsorbed by the mucous membranes of the small intestine and colon.

The stools carry no more than 120 grams of water with them when they exit the body. Of the 7 liters of water provided to produce the digestive juices, 6.88 liters (or 97 percent of the total volume) is reabsorbed by the intestinal mucous membranes and fed into the blood so that it can be reutilized elsewhere in the body. In reality, the reabsorption by the digestive tract is higher. It carries not only the 6.88 liters of digestive juices brought there every day, but also the 1.2 liters of water that is drunk directly and the liter of water that comes in bound to foods.

TABLE 2.4. HYDRIC BALANCE SHEET OF THE DIGESTIVE TRACT (AVERAGE, IN LITERS)

INTAKE	
Bound water	1.0
Drinks	1.2
Saliva	1.0
Gastric juices	1.5
Pancreatic juices	0.75
Bile	0.75
Intestinal juices	3.0
Total	9.2
OUTPUT	
Water in the stools	0.1
Reabsorbed water	9.1
Total	9.2

Kidneys

The filtering of toxins by the kidneys entails the removal of about 4 ounces (120 milliliters) of water per minute. Over a twenty-four-hour period, this amounts to some 180 liters of water removed from the blood. Obviously we do not eliminate 180 liters of urine on a daily basis, but only 1 to 2 liters. What becomes of the other 178 liters? It is reabsorbed into a special part of the kidneys (the convoluted tubules), from where it is fed back into the bloodstream. Thanks to this mechanism, the body avoids the loss of the quantity of water that must be removed to purify the blood—a quantity too great to be easily replaced by the ingestion of a new supply from outside the body.

Here again we can see the body's wonderful ability to adapt. To survive with a limited liquid intake, it exploits the water it has at its disposal by ceaselessly circulating it from one part of the body to another, where the same water can perform a large number of different tasks.

3

The Harm Caused by Dehydration

Our bodies are constantly dealing with liquid deficiencies.

Every day we expel 2.5 liters of water from our bodies in the form of urine, sweat, water vapor from the lungs, and the liquid contained in stools. When an equivalent intake of water is maintained, the body's hydric budget is in balance. Conversely, if the liquid intake is insufficient, this balance sheet goes into the red, and the process of dehydration begins.

The dehydration of the body can occur quite quickly. Although human beings can survive for a fairly long period without food (more than six weeks, as is shown by certain therapeutic fasts), the same does not hold true for going without liquid. Three days without any liquid, either in the form of drinks or what is bound to solid food, is sufficient to create serious physical breakdowns. Two or three days longer is fatal.

Since we usually have enough water at our disposal to meet our needs, we give no thought to just how long we can do without water and, consequently, just how short is the path that leads to dehydration and death.

TABLE 3.1. DAILY HYDRIC BALANCE SHEET
(AVERAGE, IN LITERS)

WATER ABSORPTION	
Water from drinks	1.2
Water from foods	1.0
Metabolic fluid	0.3
Total	2.5

WATER ELIMINATION	
Urine	1.5
Sweat	0.5
Through the lungs	0.4
Through the intestines	0.1
Total	2.5

Serious problems due to dehydration commence when loss of weight caused by loss of water reaches approximately 10 percent of total body weight. Death occurs when weight loss reaches about 20 percent. For a person weighing 160 pounds, this would mean a loss of 16 and 32 pounds (approximately 7 and 14.5 liters), respectively. As humans eliminate around 6 pounds (2.5 liters) of liquid a day, they would effectively reach these critical thresholds at the end of three and six days without water.

There is a margin of error, however. When the body is no longer receiving water, it does not continue to eliminate 2.5 liters of liquid a day but reduces the volume expelled. This ensures that serious problems and death do not occur until two or three days later. The longest cases we know of survival without water, however, do not exceed ten days.

These percentages are equally valid for the majority of animals. There are two notable exceptions: camels, who can endure a water loss equivalent to 30 percent of their weight (hence their tolerance of the hostile desert environment); and chameleons, for whom water loss can go as high as 46 percent of their weight.

So what precisely happens when the body is deprived of liquids over a long period?

First, blood volume tends to shrink, surrendering part of its own constituent water to the kidneys, the sudoriferous glands, and the other excretory organs that remove toxins from the body. But a great reduction in blood volume eventually causes loss of consciousness, as well as problems supplying the cells with the oxygen and nutrients they need.

It is therefore necessary for the body to adjust. As it is no longer receiving water from external sources, it must draw what it needs from the nearest internal source: the extracellular fluid. Unfortunately, this withdrawal means that the cells are no longer surrounded by a sufficient quantity of liquid, and this degrades their functioning so it is intermittent and incomplete.

The situation cannot help but continue to deteriorate, because the blood continues to give an uninterrupted supply of liquid to the excretory organs, forcing the interstitial compartment to give up its water. This reduction of interstitial liquid cannot go on for long without generating new disorders. The thickened interstitial fluid is no longer capable of ensuring that the exchanges between the blood and the cells take place as they should.

To remedy this, the body is again forced to find another solution and begins to draw liquid from the intracellular fluid, withdrawing water the cells normally use when it's available but can do without if need be. But the rest of their water is indispensable, and if the cells were forced to give it up, this would compromise their ability to function. If the body still does not obtain water from an external source, after taking all the other adaptive measures described, it draws water from this deep level of the body. The water content of the cells must then shrink, as the body has no other additional area from which it can withdraw water.

Once the deepest level from which the body can draw water has been reached, the withdrawals are reapportioned among the three levels, with the most being taken from the area that is richest in water. The level that is most greatly affected by a lack of water is consequently the cellular level, which contains 70 percent of the water in the body, versus 22.5 percent at the extracellular level and 7.5 percent at the blood level.

Overall dehydration of the body engenders two serious metabolic problems that are the main causes of all the various disorders caused by dehydration: enzymatic slowdown and autointoxication (poisoning by toxins produced within the body).

ENZYMATIC SLOWDOWN

The role of enzymes is to perform the many biochemical transformations necessary for the body to function. To do this they need, among other things, an environment richly supplied with water. The more the environment in which the enzymes act is encumbered by other enzymes, and also by the substances on which they work or that are created by their activity, the more difficult it is for the enzymes to perform their tasks correctly. They are least efficient when body fluids are thick and concentrated—in other words, when the fluids are more viscous. It so happens that higher viscosity is the inevitable result of dehydration.

When the volume of blood and cellular fluids shrinks, the substances normally held in suspension in them become more tightly packed. The body fluids become more highly concentrated, thus giving the enzymes an environment poorly suited for their activity, a situation that continues to deteriorate as long as dehydration remains an issue.

At first, the enzymes continue to work, but at a slower pace. Later, this rhythm slows further, and the biochemical transformations become intermittent and incomplete. Finally, they cease altogether because of the overly high viscosity of their environment. Death inevitably ensues following this development.

Enzymatic slowdown eventually paralyzes all the body's activity, as the production of energy, hormones, reparative substances, and so on necessary for the body to perform properly gradually decreases.

The influence of dehydration on physical abilities has been calculated to a very precise degree in sports medicine. The figures supplied by this research clearly show the speed with which dehydration has an effect on body function. A loss of liquid equivalent to 1 percent of total body weight is enough to diminish the body's working capacity by 10 percent. At a 2 percent loss, this capacity becomes 20 percent less efficient. The reduction in effectiveness continues at the same pace until around 10 percent, the stage at which the dehydrated individual loses consciousness, along with all motor and physical effectiveness. Beyond this point, the physical breakdown only increases, leading ultimately to death.

For a person weighing 160 pounds, 1 percent of body weight is equal to 1.6 pounds, or 0.7 liter of water, a quantity that is easily lost through the sweat caused by one hour of physical exercise at an ambient temperature of 64 degrees Fahrenheit (18 degrees Celsius). At 82 degrees Fahrenheit, the hydric loss borders on 3 liters an hour, equaling more than 4 percent of total body weight and a 40 percent loss in physical ability.

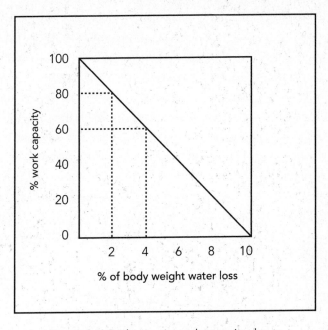

Figure 3.1. Reduction in work capacity due to dehydration (based on L. Hermansen, cited in Alain Garnier, *Alimentation et sport*)

AUTOINTOXICATION

Every day, cells produce wastes and metabolic residues. The essential support medium for evacuating wastes is water: sweat is composed of 99 percent water; urine, 95 percent; and exhaled air and stools, 80 percent.

When the body does not have the liquids it needs to perform its functions properly, elimination continues, but with a reduced quantity of water. Urination is less frequent and the urine is thicker; sweat is more concentrated; and stools are dry and hard. Under these conditions, toxins are eliminated at a reduced rate. Waste products accumulate in the excretory organs, are deposited on the walls of the vessels, and congest the organs. The content of toxins in the blood and cellular fluids increases. All these factors contribute to the autointoxication of the body, which is considered in holistic medicine as the starting point for every illness.

The situation can deteriorate even further. When the body has been deprived of liquids for a long time, eventually there is not enough liquid to eliminate the toxins the body continues to produce. The toxins then become concentrated *inside* the body. At this point, the body begins to suffocate in its own wastes; cellular activity comes to a halt, and death follows.

These two situations, enzymatic slowdown and auto-intoxication, engender all the disorders characteristic of dehydration.

ACUTE AND
CHRONIC DEHYDRATION

Most people don't think they need to worry about dehydration. To them, dehydration is something that happens to travelers in the desert when they run out of water.

But there is a chronic form of dehydration that does not have the sudden and intense nature of the acute form. *Chronic dehydration is widespread in the present day and affects everyone who is not drinking enough liquid.*

The troubles that result from chronic dehydration are not as pronounced as those created by the acute form. The liquid loss is always less than the 10 percent of body weight cited earlier as the cause of serious physical problems that can threaten a person's survival.

Chronic dehydration is not severe enough to result in death or serious illness, but it is enough to cause numerous functional and lesional disorders that are more or less irritating or painful. These disorders are many and varied, because the lack of water brings about a general weakening of the body's internal cellular environment. Of course, the weakest organs give way first, and that is where the disorders appear.

In the next section, several examples are given of the health problems that can result from chronic dehydration of the tissues. These problems can have a variety of different causes, but dehydration is a possible cause of each one.

HEALTH PROBLEMS THAT CAN BE CAUSED BY CHRONIC DEHYDRATION

Fatigue, Energy Loss

Dehydration of the tissues causes enzymatic activity to slow down, even for enzymes active in the production of energy. This production can fall so low in the case of acute dehydration that the individual suffering from it may not even be capable of standing up. He or she remains prostrate and motionless, in a somnolent or even unconscious state.

Although it does not go to this extreme, chronic dehydration nonetheless engenders a sense of chronic fatigue and lassitude. The effect on a person's psychic state is a noticeable lack of enthusiasm while working and a loss of joy in living.

If a person in this situation starts drinking sufficient quantities of water again (the question of quantity is discussed in chapter 6), his or her energy returns. A generous intake of water retriggers enzymatic activity, hence the return of energy. Regaining strength and energy is one of the effects mentioned by the majority of people who increase their water consumption to bring it back to normal levels.

Constipation

When an alimentary bolus (a mass of chewed food) enters the colon, it contains too much liquid to allow stools to form properly. The excess water is absorbed by the wall of the colon to reduce this content. The removal process continues until the stools acquire their normal consistency, which allows easy evacuation.

With chronic dehydration, however, the removal of liquid can be excessive. As the body is not receiving enough water from the outside, it seeks to obtain it from all possible sources. One of the means it has available is to withdraw water from one part of the body to put it at the disposal of another. In this case, the body withdraws more water from the stools than it would normally. They then become dry and hard and difficult to eliminate.

Constipation caused by chronic dehydration can be corrected only by increasing daily water consumption. The body then ceases to make extra withdrawals of water from the stools, and they regain the necessary moisture to be eliminated normally.

Digestive Disorders

Various digestive disorders can be caused by a lack of water: poor digestion, gas, bloating, pain, nausea, indigestion, and loss of appetite. In fact, the body produces 7 liters of digestive juices daily. In the event of chronic dehydration, the secretions are less abundant, and the digestive process cannot perform properly.

In this case, water should not be consumed during meals but separately, throughout the day, especially thirty minutes before mealtime. An amount of 10 ounces or 3 deciliters at a time would be appropriate. Drinking throughout the day and before meals ensures that the quantity of water available for the production of digestive juices is sufficient.

High and Low Blood Pressure

The body's blood volume is not enough to completely fill the entire set of arteries, veins, and capillaries. Regions of the body in which requirements for blood are not very high will therefore supply some of it to regions whose needs are greater.

For example, when we eat, the digestive tract has a greater need to be well irrigated than the muscles of the legs, which are idle at the time. The blood vessels of the legs therefore contract and expel some of their blood toward the vessels of the digestive tract. These vessels then dilate to take in the extra blood they need. The vasoconstricting and vasodilating capabilities of the vessels allow the body to make adjustments that are crucial for its proper functioning.

However, these capabilities can be used in exaggerated ways, which can result in health problems. Among other things, when the body deals with too little blood volume caused by chronic dehydration, the blood vessels sharply contract. This ensures that the volume of blood available—already limited in normal circumstances, but now even more so because of dehydration—sufficiently fills the vessels without leaving free spaces where pockets of gas could form.

But this defensive vasoconstriction can become permanent if the body is suffering from a chronic liquid deficiency, and the result is chronic high blood pressure. The increase of tension in the walls of the veins is exacerbated by a rise in blood viscosity. The body is compelled to raise the pressure with which it pushes the blood through the veins to compensate for the slowdown in circulation caused by the increased thickness of the blood.

While dehydration can in some cases be responsible for high blood pressure, it can also encourage the opposite condition, low blood pressure. If hypertension is characteristic of people whose vessels have good tone and contract easily, low blood pressure afflicts those whose vasoconstricting capabilities are weak. Their blood pressure is lower than average because their blood is circulating though vessels that are not tight and narrow.

When a person with low blood pressure becomes dehydrated, the blood volume shrinks, but the vessels cannot reduce their diameter sufficiently to compensate for the lower blood volume. The blood is thus circulating in slack, poorly filled vessels, and the pressure falls even lower.

Quite logically, then, an increased consumption of water is one of the keys to treating both health problems.

Those with high blood pressure should drink more to bring the blood volume back to normal and allow the vessels to abandon their state of chronic defensive vasoconstriction. Of course, the consumption of water should be increased gradually by spacing drinks out over the course of the day, to avoid overtaxing the heart or the vessels.

Those suffering from low blood pressure need the additional water intake to compensate for the weakness of the vasoconstricting capabilities of the vessels. If they are amply filled with blood, they do not have to contract as much.

Gastritis, Stomach Ulcers

To protect its mucous membranes from being destroyed by the acidic digestive fluid it produces, the stomach secretes a layer of mucus. This mucus is composed of 98 percent water and 2 percent sodium bicarbonate (the same chemical compound as baking soda). The large quantity of water forms a thick barrier between the mucous membranes and the acids of the gastric juices. Because of its alkaline properties, the bicarbonate that permeates the mucus also neutralizes the acids that attempt to cross this protective barrier.

In a state of chronic dehydration, the stomach does not have enough liquid available to properly manufacture the mucus. Among people who are predisposed to these kinds of disorders, some zones of the stomach do not have a good lining of mucus and thus are poorly protected. These zones can be attacked by the acids, which first cause an inflammation of the mucous membrane (gastritis), then lesions (ulcers).

In such cases, rather than resorting to artificial palliatives, it is preferable to assist the body to produce its own palliative, or protective mucus, by drinking more. A fairly generous consumption of water helps the stomach again produce sufficient amounts of mucus so it can protect its walls from attack.

According to the research of Dr. Fereydoon Batmanghelidj cited in his book *Your Body's Many Cries for Water*—and practice has confirmed this in numerous cases—even the acute crises and pains caused by gastric ulcers (if not perforated) are quickly soothed by drinking an abundant amount of water. Emergency treatment consists of drinking a liter or so of water.

Here is an extract from his book that perfectly illustrates his position:

> Late one night . . . Dr. Batmanghelidj discovered the medicinal value of water in disease when, in place of medications he did not possess at the time, he had to prescribe two glasses of water to an ulcer patient in extremely severe abdominal pain. Within eight minutes the pain disappeared, and according to him, a new era in the advancement of medical science was born. For the next 25 months he became completely engrossed in clinical research of the medicinal values of water in stress reduction, and treatment of stress-related disease conditions of the body in Evin prison, "a most ideal stress laboratory." (pp. 179–80)

Respiratory Troubles

The mucous membranes of the respiratory region are slightly moist to protect the respiratory tract from substances that might be present in inhaled air (dust, pollen, and so on) but also to make the air more humid when it is too dry. If the body lacks water, portions of the respiratory mucous membranes dry out; they become less permeable to gaseous exchange and more sensitive to external attack. The result is a propensity for coughs and breathing disorders that vanishes once the body is properly rehydrated.

Acid–Alkaline Imbalance

For the body to function at its best, there should be a balance internally between acid and alkaline substances. The current lifestyle and diet of most people have a tendency to acidify the internal cellular environment of the body; numerous health problems can result. (For more on this topic, see my book *The Acid–Alkaline Diet for Optimum Health*.) This acidification is made worse by insufficient consumption of water.

The primary reason is that the enzymatic slowdown caused by dehydration prevents biochemical transformations from taking place properly. Instead of being carried through to completion, they are interrupted at various intermediary stages during which the substances being transformed are most often in an acid state. Internal production of acids exacerbates the acid intake from external sources, which is high in the modern diet overloaded with protein and carbohydrates.

The acidification of the body's internal cellular environment can also be reinforced by a water deficiency, because the excretory organs responsible for the elimination of liquids (the skin and kidneys) also rid the body of acids. A reduction in the volume of urine and sweat thereby reduces the evacuation of acids.

Excess Weight and Obesity

Those who are overweight are eating more than their bodies are capable of using and eliminating. But why do we have a tendency to eat more than our physiology needs? There are numerous possible reasons, but one of them—thirst—is rarely mentioned.

There are two ways to satisfy thirst: we can drink a lot of fluids, or we can eat foods rich in water. If we opt for the second solution, the body receives the liquids it needs, but it also takes in nutritive substances it doesn't need, which contribute to increased weight. More often than we might think, when we are thirsty we make the mistake of eating rather than drinking.

Although the two sensations are distinct, thirst is often confused with hunger. One reason is that eating can soothe thirst. A second reason is that the fatigue that accompanies dehydration is wrongly interpreted as a lack of energetic fuel, that is, sugar. In both cases we are dealing with a false sensation of hunger.

When we confuse thirst and hunger, a vicious circle is rapidly generated, because the more we eat, the greater is our need for water with which to manufacture digestive juices. So the more we eat, the thirstier we become. And because we are already confusing the sensation of thirst with that of hunger, we again eat instead of drink, which only increases our need for water, which is again mistakenly interpreted as hunger.

To break this vicious circle and reduce the quantity of food ingested, water consumption must be considerably increased. If we drink much more than we normally would (more than 2 liters a day), these false sensations of hunger cease. The quantity of food consumed shrinks and adjusts to the body's needs.

In addition to the beneficial effect of reduced food intake, an overall stimulation of metabolic processes occurs. This is because the rehydration of the tissues retriggers enzymatic activity, and thus the combustion of excess fat as well.

Eczema

The sudoriferous glands eliminate on a daily basis some 20 to 24 ounces (6 to 7 deciliters) of sweat, the amount necessary to dilute toxins so they do not irritate the skin.

In a state of chronic dehydration, however, the liquid volume available to create sweat is insufficient. The sweat becomes more concentrated and aggressive as a consequence, resulting in irritation and inflammation of the skin, red patches, itching, and various kinds of pimples and microlesions.

Since sweat transports the same kinds of toxins as urine, increased consumption of water is doubly beneficial: the toxins diluted in a larger quantity of sweat cease to have such a destructive effect on the skin, and the surplus water increases the renal elimination of toxins, thus shrinking the amount that makes its way to the skin.

Cholesterol

Cholesterol is one of the body's most useful substances. It is harmful only when present in excessive amounts, and then its greatest threat is to the circulatory system.

Out of the total quantity of cholesterol found in our bodies, one-third comes from food, and the body produces two-thirds. This production takes place in the liver and intestines. Hypercholesterolemia, the medical term for excessive cholesterol in the blood, can therefore have either an external cause (the foods we eat) or an internal cause (endogenous overproduction).

Among the numerous functions it performs, cholesterol takes part in the construction of the membranes (or walls) of the cells. Its role consists primarily of making them impermeable. The cells' need for cholesterol is constant, so the body produces it constantly. But this production can become excessive under certain circumstances and lead to hypercholesterolemia. This is notably the case with dehydration.

How does this occur?

When dehydration causes too much liquid to be removed from inside the cells, the body tries to stop this loss by producing more cholesterol. A higher level of cholesterol effectively enables the cellular membrane to become less permeable, which in turn prevents too much fluid loss. But while this overproduction remedies the ill effects of dehydration, it also has the negative consequence of increasing the cholesterol in the bloodstream.

In such cases, regular consumption of abundant water limits the production of cholesterol. This can be accomplished with no change in diet, because food is not the cause of the overproduction.

Cystitis, Urinary Infections

The harmful influence of liquid deficiency is well known in connection with urinary infections. If the toxins contained in urine are insufficiently diluted, they attack the urinary mucous membranes and create microlesions. These lesions then form entranceways for germs, which settle in the membranes, multiply, and engender painful infections.

Drinking large amounts of water to dilute the urine and ensure that the germs are carried away is thus perfectly justified. But the water also intervenes in another way. The microbes responsible for urinary infections often originate in the intestines. They are microorganisms of the intestinal flora that were originally beneficial, but then mutate and become virulent when intestinal transit is too slow. Subsequently migrating elsewhere in the body, among other destinations toward the nearby urinary tract, these microbes engender infections.

An increased consumption of liquid is thus not only beneficial in the urinary tract, but also at the starting gate for infections—the intestinal milieu (for example, by preventing constipation).

Rheumatism

Joints become inflamed and painful when they are attacked by irritating substances, which are usually toxins produced by the body itself. These pains increase in proportion to the concentration of the toxins. Dehydration abnormally increases the concentration of toxins in the blood and cellular fluids, enhancing their ability to act as irritants. The pains of rheumatism should therefore be soothed or suppressed by increasing the amount of water ingested daily.

Such a therapy is often effective for several reasons: ingesting more water reduces the concentration of toxins in body fluids; toxins are more easily eliminated when there is more water available; and rehydration of the tissues has beneficial effects on the joint cartilage.

Cartilage tissue has a very high water content. Its role is to protect the contact surfaces of the bony pieces of the joint. Thanks to the cartilage, these bony pieces can slide over one another without being damaged. But when the body is suffering from chronic dehydration, the cartilage grows thinner, and the bones start rubbing together. The resulting irritation, added to that caused by the toxins, inflames the joint and causes intense pain. The rehydration of the cartilage is therefore one of the beneficial effects of treating rheumatism by increasing the consumption of water.

Premature Aging

The normal aging process involves a gradual loss of volume of the extracellular and intracellular fluids. As we saw earlier, the body of a newborn child is composed of 80 percent liquid, but this percentage declines to no more than 70 percent in an adult and continues to decline with age. This water loss contributes to the slowing down of exchanges and the loss of volume in the flesh that are characteristic of natural aging.

However, loss of water in the tissues can be intensified and accelerated when the liquid ingested on a daily basis is not enough to meet the body's needs. Older people who do not drink enough aggravate the normal dehydration process that accompanies natural aging. They age much more quickly than necessary, simply because of poor hygiene.

Drinking enough liquid is essential throughout life. Unfortunately, the elderly often do not drink enough, perhaps because they do not always clearly perceive the sensation of thirst.

⤳

To avoid dehydration, the body pushes us to drink by triggering a disagreeable sensation: thirst. Theoretically, it should therefore not be possible to become dehydrated. And yet the fact remains that many people do not drink enough.

So just what is thirst? When and how does it occur? Why don't we always understand what it is telling us? These are a few of the questions touched on in the next chapter.

4

Thirst

The body uses the sensation of thirst to avoid dehydration. It is an alarm signal that goes off every time the body begins to experience a lack of water. Thirst compels us not only to drink, but to drink as much as is necessary to correct the hydric imbalance.

The sensation of thirst is proportionate to the deficit. It is slight if the body's water deficiency is limited; it is intense if the lack of water is substantial. If not quenched, thirst increases with time because even when the body lacks enough water, it continues to lose water in the elimination of toxins and the regulation of temperature (via perspiration).

Thirst manifests in the mouth. It is characterized by dryness and a disagreeable constricting sensation of the pharynx, glottis, and tongue.

Once a person has drunk sufficient liquid to remedy the deficit, the sensation of thirst disappears. Until this deficit has been filled, even considerable consumption of water in a very short time does not prompt diuresis (increased excretion of urine), as it would in normal circumstances. Diuresis occurs only after more water has been ingested than required by the body to meet its needs.

As a significant deficiency of liquid rapidly has fatal consequences, the sensation of thirst grows more imperative the greater the deficiency. It becomes a demand that, under normal circumstances, continues until the individual has drunk.

Although it seems that thirst always manifests in the same way, two different kinds of thirst can be distinguished, depending on where in the body the hydric deficit is most severe: extracellular (or hypovolemic) thirst and intracellular (or osmotic) thirst.

EXTRACELLULAR THIRST

Extracellular or hypovolemic thirst manifests when the volume of blood and extracellular fluid becomes too low (*hypo* means "low" and *volemic* means "volume"). The purpose of this thirst is to compel rapid intake of water to bring the volume of blood and extracellular fluid back to normal, preventing the body from drawing more water out of the cells. The latter solution can be damaging physiologically, whereas the simple consumption of water is not.

At first glance, extracellular thirst could appear to be due solely to the loss of liquids engendered by the activity of the eliminatory organs. Although the blood and extracellular fluid guide toxins to the kidneys and the skin, and also supply the water these organs need to create urine and sweat, these liquid losses are not sufficient to explain the appearance of thirst, because the need to drink does not arise every time a person urinates, or because of the perspiration caused by a normal day's activity.

Certainly, these eliminations are responsible for water losses, but because they are gradual, they can be entirely compensated for by daily consumption of liquids without inducing extracellular thirst. For this kind of thirst, another condition is necessary: the elimination of a large quantity of liquid must be accompanied by the loss of a large quantity of salt.

The salt in the body is primarily found in the blood and extracellular fluid. There is practically none inside the cells. The salt's role is the retention of water: 1 gram of salt retains 11 grams of water. Salt prevents the liquid environment in which the cells are immersed from shrinking too drastically, endangering their survival.

Salt is part of the body's defense system because it fights dehydration. Only in extreme conditions does salt leave the body in abnormally elevated quantities, such as when copious amounts of sweat are produced—for example, during a long stay in a very hot region, during a high fever, or during intense and prolonged athletic activity. Heavy sweating expels a great deal of salt from the body (except among athletes, whose bodies, accustomed to sweating regularly and copiously, take preventive measures to stem the loss). The more salt the body loses, the less water it can retain; and the less water it retains, the more it loses, and the more quickly it dehydrates.

Substantial salt loss can also occur with vomiting and persistent diarrhea.

When extracellular thirst is caused by the loss of salt and liquid, the resulting hydric deficiency cannot be corrected by simply drinking water, for two reasons.

First, the salt remaining at the extracellular level is only enough to retain the liquid still there. Any additional liquid intake, no matter how generous, would be useless, as the salt necessary to keep it there is missing. Second, consuming only water does nothing but worsen all the problems that the hydric deficiency has caused. Because of the salt loss, the saline con-

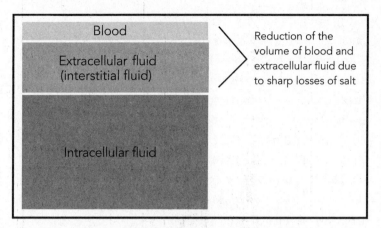

Figure 4.1. Extracellular (hypovolemic) thirst

centration of the blood and extracellular fluid has already been sharply reduced. Drinking without consuming any salt further weakens this concentration.

Only the simultaneous consumption of salt and water is capable of remedying this situation: water to reestablish the correct fluid volume, salt to retain the water ingested. A person affected by heatstroke (or sunstroke, if the cause is long exposure to the sun) gets worse if given only water, but improves rapidly if a little salt is added. It is important for this water to be drunk slowly, in small sips, to avoid hydric shock.

Extracellular or hypovolemic thirst is an exceptional circumstance, at least in its acute form; intracellular or osmotic thirst is much more common.

INTRACELLULAR THIRST

Intracellular (osmotic) thirst results from hydric deficiency inside the cells.

On their own, the cells do not voluntarily part with their

water. To the contrary, they constantly seek to conserve as much as they need. When their water content is reduced, it is because the body has withdrawn water from the intracellular level—and the cells could not oppose this. Only a serious threat could bring about such extreme measures: not, as we might think, that the volume of blood and extracellular fluids has diminished too much, but that there is too high a concentration of solids in the normal volume of these fluids.

This latter situation comes about primarily from diet. Once food has been digested, the nutritive substances exit the digestive tract to enter the blood and, almost immediately afterward, the extracellular fluid. The concentration of these liquids therefore increases during a meal and rises in proportion to the amount of food eaten (the quantitative aspect) and how rich and salty the food is (qualitative aspect).

When liquid intake is not used to dilute the blood and extracellular fluid, their concentration becomes greater, along with the osmotic pressure they apply on the intracellular fluid. A transfer of liquid by osmosis then takes place, moving fluid out of the cells to restore the osmotic balance on both sides of the cellular membrane. The cells lose water, and the resulting water deficiency triggers a sensation of thirst. This thirst is called osmotic or intracellular thirst because it is the water inside the cells that is lacking.

It is easy to see that eating creates thirst. The need to drink arises quite regularly, in fact, over the course of a meal. There is nothing cultural about this phenomenon; it is physiological. It can be observed throughout the world, among both people and the majority of animal species. Rats, for example, drink 60 percent of the water they consume in the course of a day right after a meal; dogs, 90 percent of their daily ration.

Intracellular thirst can also make an appearance long after a meal. People become thirsty late at night when they

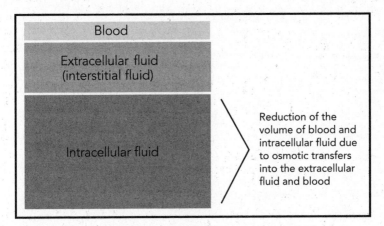

Figure 4.2. Intracellular (osmotic) thirst

are digesting their evening meal. When thirst appears at waking, it is because the excretory organs have done a poor job of purifying the blood over the course of the night. In the morning it still contains too many of the toxins it took in from the evening meal.

The interdependence of diet and thirst explains several phenomena: why heavy eaters have heavy thirsts and light eaters, light thirsts; why during a fast the sensation of thirst diminishes greatly (except when there is a sudden increase of toxins in the blood); and why desert dwellers can survive on very modest rations of water (their diet is very moderate).

Contrary to what occurs with extracellular thirst, the quenching of intracellular thirst is achieved with unsalted water, because any salt intake would only increase the already high concentration of the blood and extracellular fluid. Further, pure water more easily absorbs the toxins that need to be carried to the excretory organs than salty water.

Depending on the cause, the need to drink could involve either intracellular (the most common case) or extracellular thirst. In exceptional situations of water deprivation, the two kinds of thirst can combine.

LOSS OF THE SENSATION OF THIRST

The sensation of thirst is an alarm signal sent out by the body, so it should be perceived by everyone. But there are some people who say they are never thirsty and consequently drink very little.

There are two principal causes for loss of the sensation of thirst.

The first is the lack of reaction to the alarm signal of thirst. When a person regularly refrains from drinking, even though urged to do so by thirst, the sensation of thirst diminishes, and the disagreeable sensations of dry mouth, constriction of the pharynx, and so on are no longer felt so acutely.

The process is similar to what occurs in people who often carry hot plates, such as cooks. They do not react to the burning sensations affecting their hands, so their hands become more accustomed to the heat. Over time, they become capable of tolerating fairly high temperatures.

In the case of thirst, the person who drinks little becomes increasingly tolerant of thirst and no longer clearly perceives the alarm signal sent by the body. This is only true, however, for the sensation of thirst, and not for its consequences: these individuals inevitably suffer from chronic dehydration despite their absence of thirst.

Loss of the sensation of thirst is rare among children, relatively widespread among adults, and quite common among the elderly. The latter can have a completely dry mouth and no desire to drink, nor even the sense that they should have something to drink.

The second reason why the sensation of thirst can be lost

is confusion between thirst and hunger. As we have seen, these two sensations, although distinct, are sometimes commingled. If we regularly alleviate thirst by eating, the sensation of thirst diminishes or is not perceived for what it is.

Fortunately, like all physiological functions, the slumbering sensation of thirst can be reawakened if we force ourselves to drink normally, even when we don't feel thirsty. After several days, we will note with surprise how thirsty we are despite all we have drunk!

5

What to Drink

Throughout this book, we have been examining how the human body needs a generous intake of liquid daily to function properly and avoid dehydration. But we have not discussed which liquids. The key questions are: Are all drinks of equal value in this regard? What are the characteristics a drink should have to be physiologically beneficial?

The drink should be easily assimilated by the digestive tract and cross easily through the walls of the capillaries and cellular membranes. It should not contain any irritating factors when drunk regularly in large quantities. It should not have an unpleasant flavor, upset the digestion, overstimulate intestinal transit, have overly calming or exciting effects, and so forth. These kinds of undesirable effects could lead a person to stop consuming the liquid before the body's liquid needs have been met.

The liquid that best responds to all these imperatives is incontestably water, simple drinking water. Water is the fundamental drink of human beings because it is the one nature has specifically provided them.

WATER

Drinking water is never pure in the chemical meaning of the word. Water that is composed exclusively of two hydrogen atoms and one oxygen atom (H_2O) can be created only in the laboratory. Generally, water contains mineral salts that it has captured while traveling underground. Drinking water is not a uniform substance that always has the same composition wherever it is found. To the contrary, its mineral content and consequently its character (its taste, its odor) vary according to its provenance.

There are many different kinds of water, but they can be separated into four major groups.

1. **Odorless, tasteless waters.** These are the purest waters, whose mineral content is quite low. Evian water, for example, is the benchmark used by professionals in the bottled water industry.
2. **Odorless waters that have taste.** These are the classic spring waters. Minerals like calcium, magnesium, or sodium confer a slight flavor. The extreme example is Vichy Celestin water, which has a very pronounced salty flavor because of its high sodium content.
3. **Waters with odor and no taste.** These are also classic spring waters. In contrast to the waters of the second group, they contain minerals like sulfur that give them a strong and characteristic odor. These waters are not sold commercially but are available directly from the spring at the thermal spa.
4. **Waters that have taste and odor.** This is tap water; the presence of chlorine gives it both odor and taste.

Despite their different characteristics, all these waters can be drunk by human beings to no ill effect.

Ideally, potable water should be odorless and have no flavor, unless the flavor is quite discreet. Numerous springs supply such water. In the past, only people living near these springs could benefit from them, but today these waters are available in bottles and sold all over.

Spring water is not sufficient to cover the needs of the constantly growing population of the Earth, so waters from other sources are used. These are primarily waters from underground aquifers, rivers, and lakes. The water from these sources is not usually directly consumable; it first needs to be cleaned and disinfected. It also requires treatment to make sure it is not contaminated or altered by its prolonged stay in the pipes that carry it to its eventual consumers.

Regular tap water does not have the properties of spring water, but an effort is made to make it as similar as possible. This goal has been partially achieved, which means that in the present day water from the tap is most often of good quality. In any event, it is cleaner and healthier than the stagnant waters of the wells and cisterns our ancestors used.

Today, most human beings have two primary sources of water: tap water, and water from springs that has been bottled.*

TAP WATER

The composition of tap water varies from region to region based on its source. Its flavor and odor are excellent in some areas but not so good in others. Most often, the reason for the variation is the amount of chlorine used to disinfect it, which

---

*For more information on drinking water, see *The Drinking Water Book* by Colin Ingram.

depends on the virtues—or rather the absence of virtues—in the water as it comes from the source.

There are two ways to remedy the annoyance of overly chlorinated water.

The first involves filling a pitcher with tap water, then placing it inside the refrigerator for at least a quarter of an hour. The chlorine the water contains evaporates into the air, and the water loses its odor and acquires a sweeter and more pleasant flavor. This procedure is commonly used in restaurants that offer carafes of water to their customers.

The second procedure for eliminating chlorine (and other undesirable substances like lead, nitrates, and so on) is the use of filters. Today's consumers have a number of different models available to them.

Depending on the quality of the filter, the water is more or less completely stripped of all foreign substances. The taste and odor of the water obtained by these means varies greatly based on the filter used.

Except for situations in which tap water is known to contain harmful substances (heavy metals, organic wastes, byproducts of pollution), it is by and large completely suitable to be used as a drink, with or without filtering.

MINERAL WATERS AND SPRING WATERS

The waters sold in bottles come from springs whose qualities are known. What distinguishes them from one another is that, generally speaking, the mineral content of mineral waters is more stable and higher than that of waters from springs. Furthermore, the former are acknowledged to have therapeutic properties, whereas the latter are not.

But it is not the therapeutic aspect of these waters that concerns us here. We simply want to obtain good hydration or rehydration of the body with high-quality waters that can be drunk in large quantity because of their pleasant flavor.

Among all the waters, those that are less rich in minerals can be most easily assimilated and utilized by the body. In fact, the more a water is mineralized—or "thickened" by additional substances (coffee, sugar, cream, and so forth)—the greater the possibility of interference in the processes of assimilation and osmotic exchange. This kind of interference runs counter to our goal: the easy utilization of the liquid consumed by the body.

Water Filters

There are three principal categories:

1. Pour-through pitchers and filtering carafes. These are the simplest type of filters. They consist of two containers, one sitting on top of the other, separated by a filter. Tap water is poured into the top container, which can hold up to 2 gallons depending on the model. As it drips through the filter in a period of a few minutes, the water becomes purified. It then falls into the bottom container for eventual utilization.

These pour-through pitchers are sold by a number of companies (Bodum, Brita, Filt'eau, Kenwood, Pur, and so on). To be effective, the filter should be changed quite often and regularly (after 35 gallons is recommended). The active charcoal and, depending on the model, the resins used to hold the unwanted substances become quickly saturated and lose their filtering ability.

2. Filters mounted on the faucet. Faucet-mounted filters function according to the same principles as the pour-through filters but are more practical, as the water is purified as needed. Such filters are easily mounted onto the faucet and are normally sold with all the necessary adapters. They cost more than the pour-through pitcher filters, but the amount of water they can filter is greater, and the filtering is more effective. Many companies manufacture faucet-mounted filters (Aquanatura, Brita, Purolator, Rowenta, Wilmann, and so on). The filters in these appliances should be replaced often and regularly to preserve their effectiveness.

3. Fixed filters or "reverse osmosis" systems. Fixed filters are connected to the pipes where the water enters the plumbing system from the main, which ensures that all the water used in the house is purified. This equipment is much more complex than the above models. In addition to the standard resin and charcoal filters, these filters use a special process called "reverse osmosis." This equipment is by far the most effective, but it is also the most expensive and burdensome to install and maintain. It needs to be installed by professionals and inspected regularly by an expert. The main companies that market these kinds of filters are Cillit and Culligan, as well as some of the firms mentioned above.

It is generally believed that water ingested daily on a long-term basis should have a mineral content no higher than 500 milligrams per liter. The mineral content always appears somewhere on the label of the bottle.

Waters whose mineral content is higher than 500 milligrams should be used in moderation. Waters that are highly mineralized (more than 1,500 milligrams to a liter) should be used only on a short-term basis, as a therapeutic agent and not as a table beverage.

Table 5.2 lists table waters with the weakest mineral content levels in order of increasing mineral content. Some of these waters are not sold commercially on more than a local or regional level, which is why the region of origin is indicated. Two of the largest U.S. wholesalers for bottled water, with a huge selection of waters from all over the world, are located in Boca Raton, Florida. Contact information for these wholesalers can be found in the resources section on page 151.

TABLE 5.1
LEVELS OF MINERAL CONTENT IN WATER (MG/LITER)

Very low mineral content	1–50
Low to moderate mineral content	50–500
Average mineral content	500–1,500
High mineral content	More than 1,500

TABLE 5.2
WATERS WITH THE LOWEST MINERAL CONTENT

Name	Total Mineral Content (mg/liter)	Region of Origin
UNITED STATES		
Hawaii Water	0.005	Oahu
Rain	1.5	Utah
Thunder Mountain	8	Wyoming
Famous Premium Drinking Water	9	Texas
Sparkletts	18	California
Ice Mountain	19	Maine
SnowLine	19	Montana

Name	Total Mineral Content (mg/liter)	Region of Origin
UNITED STATES (CONTINUED)		
Ozardar	23	Texas
Great Bear	24	New York
Snow Valley	29	Pennsylvania
Arbutus	31–61	New York (Long Island)
Ozarka	32	Texas
Fountainhead	55	South Carolina
Lauré Pristiné Spring Water	55	Tennessee (Smoky Mountains)
Mount Olympus	56	Utah
Odwalla	60	California (Sierras)
Hawaiian Springs Natural Water	64	Hawaii
English Mountain	68	Tennessee
Eldorado Artesian Spring Water	70	Colorado
Alaska Chill	71	Alaska
Grand Springs	75	Virginia
EartH2O	78	Oregon
Cobb Mountain	80	California (northern)
Deer Park	90	Maryland
Palomar Mountain Spring Water	93	California (southern)
Colorado Crystal	95	Colorado
Loon Country	120	Maine
Arrowhead	121	California (southern)
Seven Creeks Spring Water	124	Ohio
Calistoga Mountain Spring Water	130	California
Hinkley & Schmitt	150	California (southern)
Avita	160	Michigan
Thundr Rock	160	Alabama
Crystal Geyser Natural Spring Water	165	California
Diamond Natural Spring Water	170	Arkansas (Hot Springs)
Keeper Springs	170	Vermont
Vermont Pure	170	Vermont
Deep Rock	180	Colorado
Zephyrhills	185	Florida
Trinity Springs	195	Idaho

Name	Total Mineral Content (mg/liter)	Region of Origin
UNITED STATES (CONTINUED)		
Hillcrest Spring Water	210	Wyoming
Mountain Valley Spring	230	Arkansas
Quibell	270	West Virginia
Yellowstone Headwaters	310	Wyoming
Saratoga Springs	320	New York
Adobe Springs	364	California
Noah's California Spring Water	380	San Antonio Valley
Giant Springs	414	Montana
CANADA		
Ice Age	4	British Columbia
Arctic Glacier	10	British Columbia
Spirit Water	10	British Columbia
Sugarloaf Spring Rain	23	Nova Scotia
Sun Spring Eau de Glacier	40	British Columbia
Whistler Water Pure Glacial Spring	48	British Columbia
Arctic Chiller	58	British Columbia
Royal Mountain National Springs	58	New Brunswick
Monashee	81	British Columbia
Esker	84.8	Quebec
Sparta	98	Ontario
Davren Springs	110	Manitoba
West Best Natural Spring Water	112	British Columbia
Northern Crystal	160	Quebec
Rocky Mountain Spring	165	Alberta
Naya (Mirabel)	200	Quebec
Naya (Revelstoke)	210	British Columbia
Empress Springs	235	Saanich Peninsula
Cedar Springs	236	Ontario (Oro Mountain)
Naya (Saint André Est)	240	Quebec
Canoe Springs	250	Ontario
Labrador	250	Labrador
Sahara Water	298	unavailable
Kootenay Spring	426	British Columbia

Name	Total Mineral Content (mg/liter)	Region of Origin
MEXICO		
Agua Purificada Aquasystem	86	Coyoacan
BoNatura	105	Mexico City
COSTA RICA		
Alpestre Alpina	118	San José
Katadin	158	Barva
Cristal	183	Heredia
UNITED KINGDOM		
Aqua Pura	63	Cumbria
Decante	79	Wales (Conway)
Pourshins	79	Wales (Conway)
Llanllyr	84	Wales
Glencairn Spring	91	Scotland
Lowland Glen	98	Scotland
Caledonian Springs	117.2	Scotland (Glasgow)
Strathglen Spring	119	Scotland
Highland Spring	136	Scotland
Mountain Spring	140	Scotland (Perthshire)
Ty Nant	165	Wales
Wildboarclough	174	Cheshire
Glendale Spring	182	Scotland (Perthshire)
Campsie Spring	195	Scotland (Glasgow)
Brecon Carreg	198	Wales
Glen Orrin	203	Scotland
Antrim Hills	208	Northern Ireland
Tau	208	Wales
Stretto Hills	226	Shropshire
Galloway	231	Scotland
Gleneagles	235	Scotland (Perthshire)
Buxton	280	Derbyshire
Cotswold Spring	280	Bristol
Hildon	312	Hampshire
Shepley Spring	339	West Yorkshire

Name	Total Mineral Content (mg/liter)	Region of Origin
UNITED KINGDOM (CONTINUED)		
Blue Keld	340	East Yorkshire
Abbey Well	390	Northumbria
IRELAND		
Tipperary	272	Barrisoleigh
Aveta Celtic Goddess of Healing Waters	301	Oyster Haven
Ballygowan	420	County Kerry (Newcastle West)
Nash's	450	County Kerry (Newcastle West)
ICELAND		
Thorspring	36	Reykjavik
Ice Blue	57	Thorlakshofn
FRANCE		
Mont Roucous	18.1	Midi-Pyrénées
Montcalm	20	Midi-Pyrénées
Mont-Dore	27	Auvergne
Montagnes d'Arrée	36	Brittany
Charrier	37	Auvergne
Fontaine de la Reine	40	Midi-Pyrenees
Isabelle	42	Brittany
Celtic	46	Alsace
Luchon	83	Midi-Pyrenees
Volvic	109	Auvergne
Montclar	139	Provence, Alps, Côte d'Azur
Pyrénées	149	Midi-Pyrenees
Cristaline Neyrolles	185	Rhône-Alps
Valvert	201	Champagne-Ardenne
Plancoët	231	Brittany
Roche des Écrins	240	Provence, Alps, Côte d'Azur

Name	Total Mineral Content (mg/liter)	Region of Origin
FRANCE (CONTINUED)		
Pampara	252	Aquitaine
Sainte Anne des Abatilles	259	Aquitaine
Ogeu	268	Aquitaine
Cristaline Sainte Cécile	270	Provence, Alps, Côte d'Azur
Alet	290	Languedoc-Roussillon
Cristaline Sainte Cyr	300	Central France
Evian	309	Rhône-Alps
Aix	312	Rhône-Alps
Bompart	320	Poitou-Charentes
Cristaline Saint Médard	320	Aquitaine
Fontaine de Jouvence-Sail	321	Rhône-Alps
Saint Hippolyte	330	Central France
Thonon	342	Rhône-Alps
Fontel	370	Loire Valley
BELGIUM		
Spa Reine	33	Liège Province
Spa Barisart	49	Liège Province
Duke	80	Francorchamps
Spa Marie Henriette	95	Liège Province
Bru	160	Chevron
Valvert	201	Ardennes
Aquarel	208	unavailable
Spontin	240	Spontin
Ordal	288	Ranst
Presby	288	Yvoir
Val d'Aisne	320	Aisne Valley
Top Souveraine	360	Brakel
Original Grand Cru	376	Hotton sur Ourthe les Bains
Chaufontaine	385	Ardennes
Val	400	Boortmeerbeek

Name	Total Mineral Content (mg/liter)	Region of Origin
BELGIUM (CONTINUED)		
Villers Monopole	423	Villers le Gambon
Sty	443	Ottignies
Léberg	470	Roosdaal
Fertilia	480	Roosdaal
SWITZERLAND		
San Clemente	44	Castascio
Eden Dorénaz	181	Dorénaz
Arkina	347	Yverdon les Bains
Nendaz	410	Nendaz
Fontessa Elm	497	Elm
ITALY		
Lavretana	13.9	Caruzza
Amorosa	20.2	Massa Carrara
Fonte della Alpi	21.2	unavailable
Monviso	30	Turin
Fonte Santa Barbara	35.4	Cueno
San Bernardo Sorgente Rocciaviva	38	Cueno
Bernina	39.2	Lombardy
Daggio	44.5	Lombardy
Valmora	48	Aburu
Fonte della Buvere	54.3	Piedmont
Vigezzo	55.4	Piedmont
Ducale	56	Parma (Monte Zuccone)
Azzurina	57	Betulla
Santa Rita	59.5	Genoa
Sapore di Toscana	76	Tuscany
Vaia	106.2	Brescia
Dolomiti	114	Valli del Pasubia
Fiuggi	122	Rome
Monte Bianco	122	Aosta

Name	Total Mineral Content (mg/liter)	Region of Origin
ITALY (CONTINUED)		
Sant'Antonio	133	Tuscany
Acqua Panna	137	Tuscany
Bia	150	Abrau
Cavagrande	150	Mount Etna
Pradis	154	Friuli-Venezia Giulia
Nerea	163	Marche
Roccabianca	163	Sicily
Lynx	165.5	Parma
Motette	166	Perugia
Pic	190	Turin
Acquiadi Tempia	194.4	Sardinia
Pineta	194.8	Lombardy
Gerasia	195.3	Sicily
Misia	209	Perugia
Fonte Laura	211	Como
Coralba	216	Ischia
Fonte Meo	229.6	Rome
San Benedetto	250	Scorze
Angelica	275	Umbria
San Giorgio	278	Sardinia
Cottonella	282	Rieti
Fontanaccio	295.1	Lazio
Balda	298	Veneto
Gaia	313	Marche
Fente Primavera	314	Popoli
Sorgento dell'Amore	332	Calabria
Acqua Lilia	345	Potenza
Prealpi	345.6	Lombardy
Ninfa	352	Basilicata
Fonte Santa	395	Chiara
Amerino	470	Umbria

Name	Total Mineral Content (mg/liter)	Region of Origin
GERMANY		
Cool Blue	75	Nordheim Westphalia
Artesia Quelle	204	Erhendorff
Bad Harzburger	227	Bad Harzburg
Wittenseer Quelle	425	Berlin
AquaStar	430	Friedberg-Dorheim
Staatl. Bad Brückenauer	462.1	Bavaria
St. Leonhardsquelle	485	Rosenheim
AUSTRIA		
Gasteiner	170.9	Bad Gastein
Wildalp	178	Seisenteinquelle
Triple A	200	Quelle Thalheim
CZECH REPUBLIC		
Aqua Maria	290	Marienbad
SLOVAK REPUBLIC		
Cigel Spring Water	201	Bardejov
POLAND		
DEA	340.34	Polczyn Zdroj
SPAIN		
Agua de Quess	26.8	Asturias
Bezoya	27	Sierra de Guadarrama
Font D'or	128	Girona
Orotona	147	Castille
Font del Regàs	156	Girona
Les Creus	160	Girona
Mondariz	181	Mondariz
Font Vella	192	Girona
Solan de Cabras	252	Cuenca
Agua de Cañizar	256	Teruel
Fuente Sante	314	Asturias

Name	Total Mineral Content (mg/liter)	Region of Origin
PORTUGAL		
Glaciar	16	Manteigas
Aurora	19	Aurora
Fon7es	20	Covilha
Setefontes	20	Covilha
Alardo	25.4	Castelo Branco
Àgua do Marao	27	Amarante
Serra da Estrela	27	Gouveia
Nascente Salutis	30.4	Ferreira-Parede de Coura
Àgua do Fastio	33.7 +/- 4	Terras de Bouro
Serrana	44	Cabril
Castelo de Vide	274	Alentejo
AUSTRALIA		
Rain Farm	1	Queensland
Lithgow Valley	16	New South Wales
Linton Park	35	Upper Yarra Valley
Crystal Organic Water	49	Mount Grove
Glacier Water	53	Victoria
Misty Mountain Springs	60	New South Wales
Mount Seaview Spring Water	79	New South Wales
Neverfail Spring Water	79	unavailable
Deer Spring	91	Sidney
Tasmanian Highland Spring Waters	135	Huon Valley
Gigis Water	300	Victoria
Hartz Mineral Water	400	Huon Region
NEW ZEALAND		
Brightwater Ridge	64	South Island
Edge	98.6	South Island
New Zealand Crew	98.6	South Island
Virgin Kiwi	98.6	South Island
Cool Blue	123	Putururu
Eternal Water	135	Bay of Plenty

Depending on their provenance, mineral and spring waters can be either carbonated or flat, but this has no relevance to the body's hydration; the hydrating capability of water does not diminish if it is carbonated. Indeed, people who enjoy the stimulation carbonated water provides to the mucous membranes in the mouth may drink more of it. The drawback is that carbonated water cannot be drunk in big gulps, as some people like to do. These individuals may drink less if only carbonated water is available.

Whether to drink a carbonated water is primarily a question of personal taste and habit, but digestive intolerance may also be a factor. Some people cannot drink this kind of water without belching or feeling bloated, whereas others do not experience such problems.

Some people simply do not like drinking plain water, carbonated or not, and they may have trouble fulfilling the body's need for water. But since water is the only drink that nature offers human beings—and animals as well—it is not natural to dislike water; because it is not inscribed in human physiology, this tendency can be reversed by forcing oneself to drink water regularly. Just as the liking for other drinks is formed by habit and repetition, appreciation of water can be relearned simply by drinking it. Practice shows that pleasure and habit return quite speedily.

As all drinks are composed largely of water, it is generally believed that they all contribute to hydration, so what we drink should make no difference. In reality, however, this is not the case, because the components of certain drinks retard or obstruct hydration.

There are two major classes of beverages: drinks with a strong hydrating capacity (including water) and those with a weak hydrating capacity.

DRINKS WITH A STRONG ~topic~ HYDRATING CAPACITY

Water

Since water is the main subject of this book, it is mentioned here in passing only for clarity.

The hydrating capacity of water can be enhanced by adding a structuring agent. The structuring formula is composed of ionic minerals that organize and reduce the water molecules, holding them together in small clusters, to facilitate their flow through the cell membranes. (See phion Nutrition in the resources section at the end of the book to obtain further information about this structuring agent.)

Infusions

The leaves from plants such as mint, verbena, linden, balm, and so on give a pleasant aroma and flavor to the water in which they are steeped, which makes infusions (or herbal teas) a satisfying alternative for people who don't enjoy drinking plain water. Infusions are also appreciated by people who do like water but want some variety, as well as those who prefer hot drinks.

The medicinal properties of the plants do not have a negative effect on the body's assimilation of the water. This is not the case, however, if they have been sweetened (as will be seen later, in the section on commercial soft drinks), or when they are made with medicinal plants that have diuretic properties, such as birch, horsetail, dandelion, and so forth.

The water in infusions easily penetrates the body, so they do a good job of rehydrating the body—unless the plant used for the infusion has diuretic properties, which thwart rehydration by making the kidneys excrete more water. When diuretic infusions are drunk exclusively, the volume of liquid eliminated by the body is greater than that ingested. Some diuretic plants are even capable of doubling the volume of excreted water. Not only is the ingested water rapidly eliminated, but a portion of the water held in the tissues is also removed.

Because of their dehydrating properties, diuretic infusions are not for regular everyday use. They should be used only in set amounts during a limited period.

There are other medicinal plant infusions (such as alder buckthorn and senna) that should never be used for daily drinking purposes. Their stimulating or purgative effects, among others, appear too quickly for them to be drunk in sufficient quantity to meet the body's fluid needs. Most often nature shows us—in unequivocal terms—that these infusions should not be used as simple beverages: their taste and aroma are unpleasant and discourage us from drinking them in quantity.

Fruit and Vegetable Juices

The water in fruits and vegetables—their juice—is one of the liquids nature has provided for hydrating our bodies. Juice is water bound to a substance.

Although juice that has been mechanically extracted from fruits and vegetables is easily available in great quantities, nature's original packaging suggests we should limit our consumption of pure juice to not much more than we would ingest if we ate the fruits and vegetables themselves. Most people can easily drink a 10-ounce (3-deciliter) glass of orange juice, but far fewer would want to eat at one sitting the three to four oranges necessary to create that much juice. To maintain our harmonic balance with nature and avoid taking in too high a concentration of nutrients, vitamins, minerals, sugars, and so on, we should consider juice a secondary resource, to be consumed in moderation, either pure or diluted with water.

TABLE 5.3. BEVERAGE CONTENT
(AVERAGE WATER, SUGAR, AND CALORIES PER 100 ML)

Beverage	Water (g)	Sugar (g)	Calories
Water	100	0	0
Human milk	87	7.7	76
Cow's milk	87	4.7	67
Goat's milk	87.3	6	48
Sheep's milk	82.3	4.3	103
Whey	93.3	4.7	26
Fresh-squeezed orange juice	88	11.4	49
Apple juice	86	13	53
Tomato juice	93.7	3.8	21
Black coffee	99	0.7	5
Black tea	99	0.4	2
Cocoa with milk	79	11	101
Red wine	82.5	0.15	65
White wine (sweet)	82.5	4	80
Beer	95	4	35
Soft drinks	89	12	48

DRINKS WITH A WEAK
HYDRATING CAPACITY

To say that a drink has weak hydrating capacity sounds like a paradox. Any drink is inevitably composed mostly of water, so why would it not hydrate the body? Most drinks do a good job of hydrating, but the components of some common drinks sharply reduce their hydrating ability.

Coffee, Tea, and Cocoa

Drinks that have a base of coffee, black tea, or cocoa are quite high in purines, toxins that must be eliminated from the body by urine or sweat in the form of uric acid. Purines need to be diluted in large quantities of liquid to be evacuated without irritating the mucous membranes of the kidneys and the sudoriferous glands. The consumption of coffee, black tea, and chocolate beverages brings a large quantity of water into the body, but a good portion of this water is used to eliminate the toxins these drinks also carry in.

The alkaloid content of these drinks also reduces their hydrating capacity: caffeine in coffee, theophylline in tea, and throbromine in cocoa. Among other properties, these substances raise blood pressure, which in turn increases the activity of the kidneys. The diuretic effect that results ensures that larger quantities of water than normal are removed from the blood and expelled from the body in the form of urine. Here again, the body does not profit as much from this liquid as it would from plain water.

Of course, not all the water imported by these drinks is eliminated, but the quantity from which the body benefits is reduced. Thus the hydrating capacities of these beverages are weak.

Milk

Milk is mentioned here only because many people consider it a drink. In fact, it is a food, the first food of the newborn. Although its hydrating properties for infants are undeniable, this does not mean it is a suitable beverage for an adult.

Shortly before adolescence, the stomach stops producing chymosin, also called rennin, the enzyme necessary to transform milk into a solid food (curdled milk), which can then be attacked by the digestive fluids. Milk digestion by adults is therefore frequently laborious and incomplete. For this reason, the quantity of milk we drink after a certain age should be limited.

Whey, on the other hand, is very easily digested and excellent for detoxification remedies and regenerating intestinal flora. Its laxative and diuretic properties, however, are an impediment to its regular consumption as a daily beverage. It should therefore be regarded as a supplemental drink for therapeutic purposes (see my book *The Whey Prescription*).

Commercial Soft Drinks

Soft drinks are composed of water, refined white sugar or artificial sweetener (aspartame, for example), fragrances, acids, coloring agents, and, for those with a cola base, caffeine (from the cola nut).

The soft drinks with the highest sales are those with a cola base. This means that the majority of people who quench their thirst with soft drinks do so with a beverage that, because of its caffeine content (50 mg per glass, compared to 85 mg for a cup of coffee), makes them lose water. Caffeine is a diuretic because it elevates blood pressure, increasing the rate of the production and elimination of urine.

The water consumed with these drinks therefore travels through the body too quickly. Hardly has the water entered the bloodstream than the kidneys remove a portion of the liquid and eliminate it, before it has time to make its way into the intracellular environment.

The weak hydrating capacities of commercial soft drinks also come from their high sugar content, which amounts to about 10 percent of the drink's total weight (between 70 and 120 grams per liter). In its natural state, sugar does not cause the body any problems. But the body has a much harder time properly metabolizing refined white sugar. The glucose given off by white sugar enters the bloodstream too rapidly and in too large a quantity, and the high concentration of glucose abruptly raises the osmotic pressure of the blood. To correct this imbalance, the body has to surrender water from the extracellular fluid. An unusual situation results in which the intake of a soft drink brings about a subtraction of liquid.

But the dehydrating effect of soft drinks does not stop there. The removal of extracellular fluid engenders thirst. If, in response to this thirst, another soft drink is consumed, more extracellular fluid is removed, aggravating the dehydration. Even more intense thirst results, and often another soft drink is consumed to quench it. A vicious circle is created, as the thirst is being maintained by the very beverage that is drunk with the intention of getting rid of it.

It is easy to see that soft drinks have a dehydrating effect on the body; those who drink them regularly are chronically thirsty. As their thirst is never truly quenched, they must always have something more to drink.

Alcoholic Beverages

The most obvious reason that alcoholic beverages (wine, beer, hard liquor) are not a practical means of hydrating the body is because the behavior created by the altered consciousness they induce (i.e., drunkenness) appears long before enough liquid has been absorbed to actually have a hydrating effect on the body.

Furthermore, alcohol itself has dehydrating properties, removing water from the tissues it contacts and drying them out.

Alcohol is used by cosmeticians, for example, to dry up pimples. But alcohol acts exactly the same way on the mucous membranes. When they dry out, the mucous membranes harden and lose part of their ability to assimilate substances, including water. Alcohol therefore not only increases the body's requirements for water to fight the drying of mucous membranes, it also hinders the assimilation of water by creating sclerosis in the same mucous membranes.

Alcoholic beverages are rich in various toxic substances as well, which require a great deal of water to be diluted and flushed out of the body.

Despite their high water content, alcoholic beverages are not capable of hydrating the body properly. The thirst they engender and the difficulty in quenching it are testimony to this fact.

～

As this brief examination of different drinks shows, water is the preeminent beverage for correctly hydrating the body. The major portion of the liquid drunk daily by a human being should therefore consist of water. The other drinks, even those whose hydrating properties are quite low, can certainly still be consumed, but it should be borne in mind that they cannot provide the same hydration as plain water.

6

The Body's Water Needs

What precisely are our body's needs for water? In principle, it should not be necessary to provide a numerical answer to this question. The sensation of thirst not only indicates to us when it is necessary to drink, but also—depending on the intensity of the thirst—the quantity we should drink. Our needs should always be met instinctively.

The signals the body sends to alert us of its needs are not always heeded, however. Often the quantities of water ingested are lower than our needs because our instinct to drink does not always manifest as strongly as it should. Thirst can be weakened, if not completely atrophied, in certain individuals. A precise reckoning of the hydric needs of the body is therefore useful.

Our needs are fairly easy to determine, because they are equivalent to the amount of liquid that is eliminated each day by the human body. It is imperative that the liquid lost over the course of each day be replaced by a new intake of liquid so the body does not experience a deficiency but maintains its hydric balance. But just what are the normal daily water losses of the human body? The figures can vary slightly from one study to another, but they agree sufficiently to give us a fairly precise idea of our needs.

ELIMINATIONS

As indicated in chapter 2, we eliminate some 2.5 liters of water a day. So 2.5 liters of water is also what the body must ingest to meet its needs.

This figure does not reflect the quantity of water that should be drunk, however, because the body receives liquid not only from drinks but also in the form of water bound to the solid substances of the foods we eat.

Some people's hydric needs are covered primarily by the water contained in foods and secondarily by drinks; among others the reverse is the case, and their needs are met primarily by beverages and to a lesser extent by food. In concrete terms, this would represent an intake of 1.5 liters of water from food and 1 liter from drinks, or 1 liter from food and 1.5 liters from drinks, respectively.

The average of these two figures is 1.25 liters of drinks a day. This is a fairly small quantity of liquid, amounting to six 7-ounce (2-deciliter) glasses of water. So is this all the water a body needs per day?

No, this is just an average, theoretical figure that is subject to various modifications. There are a number of factors that tend to greatly elevate these figures.

For one thing, the contemporary diet is primarily made up of dry and concentrated foods (breads, cereals, floury foods) and foods that are high in fat (meat, cold cuts, sauces, sweets, butter). A greater quantity of digestive fluids must be produced to make these foods soluble and digestible. Also, these kinds of foods can generate numerous toxins; this forces the body to surrender more liquid in order to transport waste products to the excretory organs for elimination.

But our modern diet is also three or four times saltier than it should be. Our daily need for salt is generally around 3 to 5 grams, but in practice we consume between 12 and 15 grams. Larger quantities of liquid are also necessary to dilute and eliminate this excess salt.

Where Does Excess Salt Come From?

The salt consumed by human beings comes primarily from what they add to their food:

$3/5$ is added during food production and processing
$2/5$ is added during cooking and at the table

for every 100 g	bread	500–650 mg of salt
	cheese	620–1,100 mg
	cold cuts	160–2,500 mg

Foods in the form nature offers them are low in salt

for every 100 g	vegetables	2–80 mg of salt
	fruit	1–30 mg
	cereal grains	2–10 mg
	meat	60–200 mg
	egg	95 mg
	seafood	60–150 mg
	freshwater fish	60–110 mg

And finally, as we have seen, the more we eat, the greater the body's need for liquid. Beyond the question of the quality of the food in the diet, overeating is in itself a factor in our increased water needs. We are generally taking in around 3,600 calories a day, whereas 2,100 calories are sufficient.

Water Needs and Caloric Value of Food

Under normal conditions, water needs are estimated at 1 ml per kilocalorie of food consumed for an amount higher than 2,000 kcal.

Caloric Intake (kcal)	Water Need (liters)
2,000	2.0
2,500	2.5
3,000	3.0
3,500	3.5
4,000	4.0

Observations

Average caloric consumption in different countries

France	3,633
USA	3,624
Switzerland	3,379
Japan	2,903
India	2,395

Individuals consuming the equivalent of 4,000 kcal per day should not be drinking 4 liters of water; depending on their diet, 30 to 50 percent of their water needs should be covered by the water contained in the foods they eat.

Stress is another factor that should be taken into account. Stress triggers an overall acceleration in metabolism, which makes the body produce a greater amount of sweat over the course of the day. Larger quantities of water should therefore be made available to the body, especially because the toxins created by stress require an additional intake of liquid to be eliminated.

Our current lifestyle and diet thus contribute in numerous ways to increasing our needs for water; the average figure of 1.25 liters is therefore less than what our bodies truly need. So just how much should we be drinking?

Based on a number of different studies, the daily consumption of drinks should be somewhere between 1.5 and 2.2 liters, which gives us the average figure of 1.8 liters. For the needs we are discussing, we should round that up to 2 liters (approximately half a gallon); this is the daily quantity recommended by the World Health Organization.

Two liters of liquid a day would come to about thirteen 5-ounce (1.5-deciliter) glasses, or eight 8-ounce (2.5-deciliter) glasses, or seven 10-ounce (3-deciliter) glasses a day.

But how are specific individuals to know what their own daily consumption of water should be with respect to this 2-liter figure? Should they be drinking more than this amount of liquid, or less?

MEASURING YOUR DAILY
FLUID CONSUMPTION

To determine how much you are personally drinking over the course of the day, there is only one method: measure the amount of each drink you consume. As intake can vary from one day to the next, it is a good idea to record these measurements for three or four days in succession and then take an average. It is important to record the volume measurements immediately after drinking so as not to overlook part of your daily consumption.

To begin with, determine the volume of the glass you habitually use. Check with a measuring cup if you are not sure. Then just jot down this measurement in a notebook every time you drink a glass of liquid of this size. The volume of containers that are used for commercially sold liquids (bottles, cans, cartons) is easy to determine from the label. If you regularly purchase coffee or other drinks in takeout containers, bring home an empty one of the size you usually order and measure how much liquid it contains.

Every day, add up the total volume of liquid you ingest in the form of water, infusions, and fruit and vegetable juices. Coffee, tea, chocolate drinks, and commercial soft drinks count only partially, as will beer and wine (see chapter 5). Record half their volume to give a total that is closer to the truth.

After several days, your average daily liquid consumption will appear fairly clearly. If it is below 2 liters (or half a gallon, 64 ounces), increase your daily consumption by drinking as many additional glasses of water as required to equal 2 liters. It is best to do this gradually. If your average daily consumption is already around 2 liters, continue drinking that same amount, but ask yourself if this amount of liquid truly fulfills your needs.

INDIVIDUAL NEEDS

The 2-liter figure is only an estimate of the average human being's need for water. Daily water consumption will necessarily be higher or lower depending on the individuals, their occupations, and their lifestyles.

Water needs vary from one person to the next according to weight. The daily need (ingested in the form of drink or bound water) is estimated at about ⅔ ounce per pound (40 ml per kilogram) for children and adults. Quantities of water for different weights are given in table 6.1 on page 96. For people weighing more than 220 pounds a compromise must be found between their higher needs for water and the eliminating capacities of their kidneys. A sign that the kidneys may be overburdened is edema—swelling of the legs, fingers, or eyelids.

TABLE 6.1. WATER NEEDS AND BODY WEIGHT

Weight (lb)	Water (oz)	Weight (kg)	Water (L)
40	24	20	0.8
60	37	30	1.2
80	49	40	1.6
100	61	50	2.0
120	73	55	2.2
140	85	60	2.4
150	92	65	2.6
160	98	70	2.8
170	104	75	3.0
180	110	80	3.2
190	116	85	3.4
200	122	90	3.6
210	128	95	3.8
220	134	100	4.0

People whose diet consists in large part of fruits and vegetables have slightly lower water needs because these foods bring in a great deal of liquid in the form of bound water. Increased consumption of liquid—up to 2.5 liters, sometimes more—is essential, however, for people who eat large amounts of food, who eat a high proportion of dry and salty foods, or who make their bodies more toxic by drinking large amounts of coffee or alcoholic beverages, or by smoking. The same is true for those who eat lots of meat: the greater the intake of protein, the higher the consumption of water should be.

Certain activities and life circumstances also increase the body's water needs. Following is a list of situations that, by triggering more intense periods of sweating, also cause the body to lose more water than normal:

- Athletic activities such as biking, tennis, and so on
- Walking or performing other activities under the sun, particularly in summer
- Very hot, dry weather
- Vacations or sojourns in tropical countries
- Sauna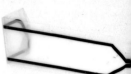
- Tanning session
- Working in overheated rooms (near a stove, for example)
- Overheated apartments or offices
- Stress, in general

How much should people drink in such situations? Heeding their instincts by drinking until thirst is satisfied should suffice for those who clearly perceive when they are thirsty. Here are some additional helpful facts:

- It is recommended that athletes drink half a liter to a full liter of water for every hour of exercise.
- During a sauna, the body perspires more than a liter of sweat in a session (40 grams a minute; 400 grams for one session of ten minutes; and 1,200 grams—that's 2.6 pounds—for three ten-minute sessions).
- To cross Death Valley on foot at a rate of eleven miles a day would require a young athlete to drink 12 liters of water a day (over 3 gallons).

When the body exerts extra effort for only a brief length of time, it is advisable to drink beforehand. When the body has to perform for a long time, as in endurance sports (e.g., bike racing, long-distance running), one should drink during and after the event. During a prolonged sojourn under the sun or in the heat, water consumption should be increased throughout the day.

One way to ensure that intake is adequately compensating for water loss is to drink until the urge to urinate manifests. After a big demand has been made on the body's hydric reserves, this need will not occur until the quantity of liquid lost has been replaced and exceeded.

WHEN TO DRINK

Are some times of the day better than others for drinking?

Generally speaking, it is a good idea to drink a large glass of water on rising, before breakfast. The body has usually not had any water for about eight hours, the only time when it goes without any liquid for so long. The body also normally eliminates a large quantity of liquid on waking: the urine it has manufactured over the night. Drinking a beverage compensates for this. Drinking water on rising also has the advantage of awakening the body. The arrival of water in the digestive tract stimulates a number of different functions.

For the remainder of the day, drink every time you feel thirsty—but be aware that thirst is not always clearly perceived.

Should you drink during meals? This is hotly debated. Some people are strongly opposed to it, but others keenly support it. What is the real story?

There is a legitimate need to drink during a meal. The intake of fluid allows better liquefaction and swallowing of dry foods and answers the osmotic thirst that is automatically triggered when you start to eat. This thirst represents the body's need for the ingestion of liquid to prevent the cells from having to cede their water to dilute the blood, which becomes thicker when it receives the nutritive substances from the meal. Drinking a beverage during meals is beneficial, because it keeps the cells from dehydrating over the long term.

Be careful that this thirst during meals remains within certain limits. If it is moderate, it is physiological, normal in all human beings as well as animals. However, if your liquid consumption is generally too restricted, the need to drink during a meal may manifest in an exaggerated manner. Because the body is chronically deficient in water, the blood does not have a sufficient volume of liquid to release for the production of digestive juices (up to 7 liters a day) nor enough volume to prevent it from becoming overly concentrated with the arrival of nutritive substances from the intestines. The need for water is therefore substantial and triggers a strong sensation of thirst that can compel you to drink a great deal during the meal.

While this fulfills the purpose of obtaining the missing liquid, annoying problems are caused by too much liquid in the digestive tract. Not only do the digestive juices have a harder time breaking down food that is drowning in water, the juices themselves are diluted and weakened. This quite naturally creates digestive disorders. Such disorders are even more likely when the beverage is not water but beer, wine, or sweetened drinks. The alcohol, tannin, acids, and sugar in these drinks have an inhibiting effect on the digestive juices.

Drinking a little water during a meal is beneficial; drinking a lot is not.

What can individuals who drink a lot of liquid during a meal do to avoid disturbing their digestion? The solution is simply to head off the demand for water by giving enough to the body *before* the meal. One half hour is a sufficient amount of time for water ingested on an empty stomach to enter the bloodstream and become available to the digestive organs (for the production of digestive juices) and the blood (to make it more fluid). Drinking a glass of water thirty minutes before a meal puts at the body's disposal a large portion of the water it will need when mealtime arrives, and less water will be drunk with the meal.

Drinking large amounts directly after a meal is obviously not beneficial and should be avoided so that digestion can occur properly. It takes an average of two hours for a meal to be digested; it is therefore advisable to limit liquid intake until then.

Of course, these are only broad guidelines. The advice to drink whenever you're thirsty remains valid. But with a little foresight, you can avoid having to deal with intense thirst at physiologically inopportune moments.

HOW TO REMEMBER TO DRINK

Some individuals get so caught up in their activities that they neglect drinking. Most often this is the result of simply forgetting, rather than not liking to drink. Nevertheless, the consequence is that the amount of water consumed per day is less than half a gallon or 2 liters.

How can we train ourselves to remember to drink? Here are three commonly used methods.

1. **Set up a schedule.** Determine in advance a timetable for drinking that is compatible with your other activities. Look for normal breaks in your schedule that are convenient and regular and which occur often enough that you will be assured of consuming a sufficient quantity of water during the day.

   Among these key moments are waking, mealtimes, breaks, arrival at work, leaving work, and returning home. If you know you will be drinking at this or that time of day every day, it will quickly become habit, fully integrated into the body's own schedule. After a while, the need to drink will begin to make itself felt at these times. It will become harder and harder to forget to drink because the habit will have become set.

2. **Prepare the amount you wish to drink in advance.** If you do not have a regular schedule or prefer not to be tied down to a timetable, instead of establishing times for drinking, establish the amount of water to be drunk during the course of the day. Calculate how much liquid you should be consuming per day in addition to what you normally drink at meals to reach a total of 2 liters or more; this is generally somewhere between 1 and 1.5 liters. Take this amount of water with you to work in bottles or a thermos and drink it whenever you wish, but make sure to finish it before the end of the day.

3. **Have a drink every time you urinate.** Drink an amount approximately equal to what has been eliminated. Initially, the association between the elimination of liquid and its replacement will spur you to drink, but over time it will become an established habit.

BIG GULPS OR SMALL SIPS?

Does it matter to the body whether you drink rapidly in large gulps or take small sips?

Physiologically, both ways (and anything in between) allow for good hydration of the body, provided the intake is sufficient. The choice of one or the other is a matter of preference. Drinking in small sips, however, has the disadvantage of making it seem prematurely as if your thirst has been quenched; the repeated contact of water with the mucous membranes in the mouth and stomach gives a false sensation of satiation. Sometimes this means the total volume of water drunk over the course of the day is insufficient to meet the body's needs. Another disadvantage is that some people acquire the habit of never drinking more than a sip or two at a time.

Drinking in large gulps is problematic primarily when the beverage is too cold. When you dump large quantities of cold liquid into the digestive tract at once, it can cause a stomach ache. When we take large gulps we also tend to swallow more air, which can lead to gas, belching, and bloating.

HOT BEVERAGES OR COLD?

A body temperature of 98.6 degrees Fahrenheit is ideal for physical function. The body is constantly striving to maintain its temperature at this level. Does this mean we should drink only beverages at this temperature? Practice tells us otherwise. Generally speaking, relative to the ideal body temperature, our drinks are either too hot (as high as 140 degrees for teas and infusions) or too cold (37 to 41 degrees for a drink taken from the refrigerator, and 68 degrees for water from the tap on a summer's day). But these gaps play a role in maintaining the ideal body temperature of 98.6 degrees.

When you are cold, hot drinks carry heat into the body and help it warm up. Conversely, when you are hot, chilled drinks allow the body to lose some of the excess heat it has stored.

One part of the exchange of calories (in the form of heat) between the body and the drinks takes place in the mouth. When a hot drink contacts the mouth's mucous membranes, the heat is transmitted to the blood. The bloodstream then carries this heat into the depths of the body and passes it on to the tissues. This process takes place quite rapidly; the temperature of an infusion, for example, drops from around 140 to 104 degrees during its journey through the mouth and esophagus.

The reverse process also takes place quite quickly. The

blood and mucous membranes actually give up enough heat to warm a chilled drink of 36 to 38 degrees to as high as 68 to 77 degrees during its brief trip from the mouth to the upper part of the digestive tract.

The speedy pace at which the temperature of the drinks changes is only possible when the quantities ingested are small, when the beverage is absorbed in small sips. In any case, drinks that are very hot or very cold cannot be drunk in large gulps; the first burns the mouth, and the latter can trigger painful constricting sensations in the stomach or even an intense headache.

If you have the habit of drinking in large gulps, be careful that the temperature of the drink is not too extreme, or the body will be incapable of moderating it while it is still in the mouth.

Paradoxically, drinking hot beverages can sometimes have a refreshing cooling effect. After exerting physical effort, the body's ambient temperature is higher than usual. The heat carried in by the beverage prompts the body to perspire. When the sweat evaporates on the skin, calories are subtracted from the body, making it feel cooler.

Although instinct serves as a reliable guide in choosing the temperature at which we drink beverages, it is still good to know the general properties, positive and negative, of cold water and hot water.

The disadvantages of hot water are minimal. When drunk plain, it does not have as pleasant a flavor as cold water. Hot water, and even more so lukewarm water, quickly create the sensation of a full stomach. The quantities drunk are consequently much less than necessary to meet the needs of the body. Water ingested in the form of plant and herbal infusions or teas (e.g., mint, verbena, linden), in contrast, goes down quite easily and in large amounts.

The primary benefit of hot water is its ability to bring heat into the body, partially relieving it of the need to produce this heat itself to maintain its normal temperature or to fight against the cold. Hot beverages (in the form of unsweetened infusions) are therefore especially beneficial for people with low energy, those who are sensitive to the cold, the elderly, or those suffering from chronic illnesses. By dilating the mucous membranes and blood vessels, hot water encourages metabolic exchanges. This is probably one of the reasons why people tend to drink hot beverages at breakfast: the heat helps the newly awakened body's "engine" get in gear.

When a person suffering from low energy drinks water that is too cold, or drinks cold water in large amounts or too hastily, this can have a chilling effect and cause the person to lose strength. Outside this situation, cold water is always beneficial.

Because of its temperature, cold water has a stimulating and vitalizing effect on the body in general. It also has a refreshing effect when the body feels hot—following strenuous physical activity, for example—and thirst is most intense, as effort has caused the body to perspire. Cold water has a pleasant flavor, and water is most often drunk at this temperature.

7

Ten Remedies for Rehydrating the Body

The best means of hydrating the body is to drink one half-gallon or more of water a day. This simple hygienic measure is the aim of the first remedy in this chapter.

The nine other proposed remedies are more therapeutic in nature.

The purpose of the two rehydration remedies is very rapid hydration of the body. They are specifically indicated for people who have a long-standing habit of not drinking enough.

The pure water remedy also hydrates the body, but its primary purpose is detoxification. It combines different natural methods for effectively eliminating toxins.

The exclusive purpose of the two dry–wet remedies is detoxification. They do not specifically hydrate the body, but they are quite useful, and they are relevant with regard to the physiological mechanisms connected with thirst discussed in chapter 4.

These are followed by two remedies that combine hydration with remineralization. In the first, the judicious choice of water brings into the body the mineral or minerals it is missing and therefore addresses its deficiencies. The second, with the help of alkaline waters (rich in alkaline minerals), contributes to the deacidification of the body, to restore the proper acid-alkaline balance.

The last two remedies concern hydration with respect to two specific fields: sports and beauty care.

These ten different remedies are within the ability of everyone to follow. Their purpose, their mode of action, and the specifics of their practice are explained so that every reader can understand how they work and how to follow them successfully. The indications are always general and broad, however. Consequently, readers should use their good sense in applying and adapting them to their specific situations and the possibilities of the moment. Some remedies may not be advisable for people with certain health conditions. As with any diet or remedy, it is best to consult a qualified health care professional before beginning. See the individual remedies for specific contraindications.

HYDRATION REMEDY

The objective of this remedy is to provide the body with the water it needs on a daily basis so that its tissues are always properly hydrated. It is not really a remedy in the true sense of the term, but a measure of standard hygiene to be followed on a permanent basis.

Method
Normal hydration of the body requires that a person drink around a half-gallon (2 liters) of water in divided doses over the course of the day.

How It Works
With regular ingestion of a sufficient amount of water throughout the day, the liquid surrendered by the blood to produce

the digestive juices, sweat, urine, and so on is always replaced immediately, and the extracellular fluid is not required to cede its water to the bloodstream. If it must do so occasionally, however, its proper volume is quickly and easily restored.

As the two higher body levels (blood and extracellular fluid) are always well supplied with water, the cells are only rarely called on to give up their fluids. They will never be dehydrated but will always be filled and surrounded by a good supply of water, which is a requirement of good health.

Water Used

Mineral water, spring water, or tap water.

Dosage

To reach the desired amount of at least one half-gallon (2 liters) of water a day, the number of times you drink depends on the volume ingested each time you drink. The number of drinks is obviously higher if you drink only a little at a time.

To space out the times you drink water during the day, follow or adapt the sample schedule below that shows the most common times when drinks are consumed. It lists nine dosage times, meaning that the amount drunk each time should be a little more than 7 ounces (2.1 deciliters), a quantity most people would have no trouble drinking in one sitting.

TIMETABLE

At waking (6 AM)	Midafternoon (3 PM)
At breakfast (7 AM)	End of the work day (5 PM)
At the start of the work day (9 AM)	At the evening meal (7 PM)
At the end of the morning (11 AM)	Midevening (9 PM)
At lunch (noon)	

Duration

As this is a method of hygiene and not a therapy, this "remedy" can be followed on a long-term basis.

REHYDRATION REMEDY #1

This first rehydration remedy aims not only to bring the body the water it needs for its normal functioning but also to fill its deeper hydric deficiencies. The person who has not drunk enough water over a long period experiences a chronic hydric deficiency, which inevitably creates a more or less substantial reduction of blood volume—and volume of extracellular and intracellular fluids. These various liquids will not regain their proper volume unless the body receives more water than it needs to meet its daily requirements.

Method

The remedy consists of drinking several ounces a day more than you normally would. If your daily needs are 2 liters, for example, you would drink 2.2 to 2.5 liters of water a day.

Note: Before using this remedy, people who have been drinking less than a half-gallon (2 liters) of water a day should take several weeks to follow—as a transitional stage—the basic Hydration Remedy discussed beginning on page 106.

How It Works

When this additional intake is drunk every day on a regular basis and consistently provides slightly more than the body needs, blood volume is constantly pushed upward and maintained at a higher level. In this way, the blood can permanently surrender some of its excess water to the extracellular fluid, which was not possible when the blood was itself lacking liquid.

Thanks to this process, the extracellular fluid regains its normal volume and even slightly exceeds it. Thus it is in a position to cede some of its excess water to the next level: the cellular level. The cells then fill their water deficiencies and regain their normal size.

This slightly excessive intake of water helps the water travel gradually deeper into the body, level by level, and properly rehydrate all its tissues.

Water Used
Mineral water, spring water, or tap water.

Dosage
Drink 2.2 to 2.5 liters a day. Use your personal timetable (see the sample given in the Hydration Remedy on page 107), but increase the amount of water drunk at each selected time to 8 to 10 ounces. Or you could continue with 7-ounce glasses and add one or two more times to take a drink of water into your regular schedule.

Duration
Tissue rehydration is a physiological process and as such does not occur instantaneously. To ensure that the water has reached the depths of the tissues and completely filled the cells, this rehydration remedy should be followed for several months.

REHYDRATION REMEDY #2

The purpose of this remedy is identical to that of the previous remedy: bring more water into the body than it needs for its daily uses so that it can easily relinquish water for the extracellular and intracellular fluids.

Method

Instead of using an arbitrary amount of water to be drunk as in Rehydration Remedy #1, this one is regulated by the body's urinations. Beyond the usual urination, the body evacuates urine every time it seeks to get rid of excess liquid. These added eliminations generally occur half an hour after you have drunk beyond your thirst (and therefore your needs).

If you drink enough water after the first urination of the morning to have to urinate again in the next half-hour, the body is experiencing an excess of liquid. This situation can be maintained throughout the day by drinking a quantity of water each time you urinate that is equal to the quantity just elimi-nated. The "too full" status is thus permanently maintained, as every loss is immediately compensated with an equivalent intake.

To keep the need to urinate from manifesting too soon after you have drunk (and consequently too often throughout the day), slightly reduce the volume of water drunk each time, being careful to ensure that it is still more than you need. This will reduce the quantity of excess liquid, so the need to urinate will be felt less often.

This gives you a certain amount of control over the num-ber of urinations.

How It Works

As the blood is receiving more water than it needs, some of this liquid travels deeper into the body, with the remainder being eliminated by the kidneys.

Water Used

Mineral water, spring water, or tap water.

Dosage

Drink as much as is necessary to maintain the rate of urinations as explained in the method section. The number of urinations will vary from one individual to the next, based on the quantity of water ingested and individual sensitivities.

Duration

Over several months, straight through or every other week.

PURE WATER HYDRATION AND DETOXIFICATION REMEDY

The objective of this remedy is to detoxify the body while hydrating it—in other words, to help it get rid of the toxins and poisons that have collected in the blood and in the extracellular and intracellular fluids. The toxins are the wastes and metabolic residues produced by the body (uric acid, urea, and so on); the poisons are contaminants coming from pollution (heavy metals such as lead or cadmium), agricultural products (e.g., insecticides), foods (additives), and so on.

Method

The remedy consists of drinking 4.2 liters (1.1 gallons) of very pure water, in seven daily doses of 20 ounces each.

How It Works

Three different factors contribute to the detoxifying action of this remedy: the purity of the water, its volume, and the forceful transit of the liquid.

PURITY OF THE WATER

Perfectly pure water consists solely of hydrogen and oxygen. Water like this would not retain its purity for long in nature;

in very short order it would become tainted with the plant, animal, and mineral substances it encountered. Indeed, water's main roles within the body are to link and transport; and water has a great capacity to absorb substances. This characteristic is what I refer to as its "snatching ability." The purer the water, the greater its snatching ability. The snatching ability of water, though, is not without limit. At a certain point, water becomes saturated and is unable to snatch anymore. This is why the snatching capacity is much weaker in impure water—its capacity to absorb is more or less completely used, the water nearing its saturation point. Pure water is used in this remedy in order to exploit this snatching property. Dr. Otoman Hanish,* who invented a similar cure, recommended the use of distilled water, which is perfectly pure water obtained from the condensation of steam. Water in the form of steam contains no foreign substances—not even minerals.

Distilled water therefore possesses very great snatching abilities—too great, in my opinion. This is why, to avoid the danger of the water's snatching minerals from the body, which would lead to severe mineral depletion, I recommend the use of water that is very low in minerals, such as that from Mt. Roucous (18 mg/liter) or Volvic (109 mg/liter). (Consult table 5.2 on pages 72–81 to find the waters with low mineral content available in your region.) This low mineral content ensures that the water is not completely pure and is therefore less likely to snatch minerals from the body. Some filters used to cleanse tap water also provide very pure waters suitable for this remedy.

When it enters the body, pure water picks up the various substances with which it comes into contact. Of all these substances, toxins are the most vulnerable to being snatched.

---

*A pioneer of natural medicine at the beginning of the twentieth century.

Because they are not part of the body, they are less firmly held in the tissues than are the substances used by the body for its own construction and maintenance.

VOLUME OF WATER

In this remedy, every time you drink (seven times a day), you consume 20 ounces (nearly 6 deciliters) of water. This water has to be drunk in as short a time as possible.

Because it enters the body in a relatively short space of time (each "dose" should not take longer than approximately thirty minutes to be consumed), this substantial volume of water creates significant variations of osmotic pressure on both sides of the mucous membranes and between the different levels of the body seven times a day. This is because the water sharply reduces the concentration of the liquid it enters (blood, for example), proportionately increasing the concentration of the liquid on the other side of the mucous membrane that separates the two liquid volumes (in the case of blood, the extracellular fluid). Also, because of the water's purity, it is even more capable of reducing the concentration than a liquid that is already laden with substances.

When the blood receives 20 ounces of water in a short time, the blood becomes much less concentrated in relation to the extracellular fluid. Although the density of the latter fluid remains stable, its level of concentration becomes proportionately much higher than that of the blood. The huge difference of concentration that results then engenders very strong osmotic pressure by the extracellular fluid on the blood.

To restore the balance of the amount of concentration, the water from the bloodstream enters the extracellular fluid (to reduce its concentration), and solid substances are transferred from the fluid into the blood (so as to raise its level of concentration). Because of the high osmotic pressure being applied, the transfers that take place in both directions are quite forceful. Numerous substances, consisting primarily of toxins that are not part of the structure of the tissues consequently leave the extracellular fluid and enter the bloodstream.

Once the water has entered the bloodstream, and then the extracellular fluid, the volume of the latter increases in size. The same process then takes place between the extracellular and intracellular fluids. As the intracellular fluid is not receiving water, its density becomes proportionately greater and creates a strong osmotic pressure. Intense osmotic transfers take place here as well: the water seeps down into the cells, and toxins arise out of the cellular depths and move into the extracellular fluid.

From every location, no matter how deeply they are placed, the toxins are gradually pulled to the surface by the play of the osmotic exchanges. The blood then carries them to the excretory organs to be flushed from the body.

FORCEFUL TRANSIT OF THE WATER

The third factor that contributes to the detoxifying properties of this remedy is the force of the liquids that course through the body, on both the superficial and deeper levels, thanks to the large volume of water being drunk. On the surface, water is rapidly eliminated, making the journey from the digestive tract into the blood and thence to the kidneys. On the deeper level, the water travels down through the body stage by stage until it reaches the cells, thanks to osmotic exchanges.

The extensive "washing" of the tissues that results cleanses the body in the same way a strong current rids the bed of a stagnant stream of what has collected there.

Water Used

Water with low levels of mineral content (see table 5.2 on pages 72–81).

Dosage

Drink a total of 4.2 liters (1.1 gallons) a day, in seven doses.

With this remedy, it is important to drink a large quantity of water at one time, so you should stick to the seven daily doses and not add additional drinking times to your schedule to reduce the quantity of each drink.

To space out these doses properly during the day, the following schedule can be used; at each of these times, drink **two** 10-ounce (3-deciliter) glasses of water.

TIMETABLE

At waking (6 or 7 AM)

After breakfast (9 AM)

Late morning (11 AM)

Early afternoon (1 PM)

Midafternoon (3 PM)

Late afternoon (5 PM)

Evening (7 or 8 PM)

Other variations are possible; it is important that the times be convenient, so you won't be tempted to skip any of them. This schedule also avoids drinking a large volume too close to bedtime so that you aren't awakened by the need to urinate and avoids drinking at mealtimes because large quantities taken during meals dilute the digestive juices and can create digestive disorders.

Note: Drinking this amount of water will reduce your appetite, so eat a modest diet while following this remedy.

To prepare the body for the demands of this remedy, establish a short transition period of two to three days to build up gradually to 4.2 liters (1.1 gallons) of water a day—for example, by drinking 10 ounces (3 deciliters) seven times the first day, 14 ounces (4 deciliters) seven times the second day, and 16 ounces (5 deciliters) seven times the third day.

Duration

For chronic problems, a three- to five-week course is required. As a general health remedy, follow for one week; or two days out of every week for one or two months.

Contraindications

Those with a weak heart or poor kidneys should not follow this remedy. People who have a tendency to retain water should make sure to check that they are eliminating as much as they ingest every day they follow this remedy. If that is not the case, they should stop the remedy.

THE DRY–WET ALTERNATION DETOXIFICATION REMEDY

This remedy aims to detoxify the body at its deepest levels, meaning to remove not just the toxins in the bloodstream but also those that are stagnating in the extracellular fluid and in the cells.

Method

The remedy consists of two phases: the first, "dry"; the second, "wet."

Dry phase: Drink nothing for 24 to 36 hours. Refrain from eating as well, or else eat only dry foods such as crackers, dried fruits, and nuts.

Wet phase: Drink 1 to 2 liters in the space of one hour to rehydrate the body suddenly and trigger a strong diuresis (increased excretion of urination). Once this has occurred, continue to drink according to the principles of Rehydration Remedy #2 (on pages 109–11) for two to three days: after every urination, drink a quantity of water equivalent to what has been eliminated to create a forceful transit of liquid through the body.

How It Works

During the dry phase, the blood is not receiving any water from outside to compensate for the losses caused by elimination. The only way it can restore its proper volume is to draw water from the extracellular fluid. Part of the water contained in this fluid then rises into the bloodstream. But this rise automatically brings about a movement of water out of the intracellular fluid to compensate for the loss of the extracellular fluid. The intensity of these movements of liquid, from the depths of the cells into the upper layers, depends on how extreme the water deficiency of the blood has become.

In tandem with this movement of liquid upward, toxins are also rising. During their travels, liquids bring with them some of the toxins they contain. These toxins are therefore compelled to climb back to the surface, which would not occur, or not so quickly and with such intensity, if this upward movement were not first artificially stimulated by the dry phase of the remedy.

The toxins that have made their way into the bloodstream have certainly left the depths, but they are still in the body; they have merely changed location. Now to get rid of them, the excretory organs have to expel them. This is where the second phase of the remedy comes in.

When you drink 1 to 2 liters of water in an hour, the blood volume climbs rapidly back to normal and beyond, which forces the kidneys to eliminate the overflow. The strong diuresis that results from the liquid assault carries the wastes out of the body with added force. By drinking after every urination, you maintain this diuresis over the entire day to ensure that all the toxins that have been unearthed are completely eliminated. The urine may be quite clear and colorless, giving the impression that few toxins are being removed. In reality, the toxins are being eliminated, but the volume of water that has been consumed dilutes the urine and removes its color.

Water Used
Mineral water, spring water, or tap water.

Dosage
Drink 1 to 2 liters during the first hour of the wet phase, then 1 large glass after every urination.

Duration
The remedy can be repeated at will, as long as a period of rest of at least three or four days occurs between remedies.

DRY–WET ALTERNATION REMEDY (SHORT VERSION)

As in the preceding remedy, the objective of this one is to force the toxins to rise from the depths of the body. It takes place, however, over a shorter period of time.

Method
A session in the sauna or physical exercise, or any other activity that causes heavy sweating, is a necessary accompaniment to this remedy.

Dry phase: Drink nothing at all during the hours preceding the activity you have selected—a sauna, for example—nor during the time you are taking the sauna or are engaged in the activity. Nor should you eat anything juicy.

Wet phase: At the end of the sauna or other sweat-inducing activity, drink 1 to 2 liters of water in one hour to trigger a strong diuresis.

How It Works

This remedy acts in the same way as the previous one. The reduction in blood volume (and the rise of toxins from the tissues it creates) is obtained by abstaining from drinking and by the very large increase of the elimination of liquids caused by the sweating session.

Water Used

Mineral water, spring water, or tap water.

Dosage

Drink 1 to 2 liters in one hour after the heavy sweating period.

Duration

This remedy can be followed on a regular basis, provided you have rehydrated fully between sessions.

HYDRATION AND REMINERALIZATION REMEDY

The purpose of this remedy is to restore mineral content to the body while also hydrating it.

Method

To follow this remedy, consume the 2 liters of water normally ingested daily, but use a spring water specifically chosen for its mineral content rather than plain tap water.

There is a huge selection of mineral waters available commercially, of both brands sold internationally and those available only regionally and sold locally.

Based on the mineral that predominates, springs are classified differently—as calcic waters, magnesium waters, sodic waters, sulfurous waters, chlorine waters, ferruginous (iron-laden) waters, and so on. These classifications are generally awarded only if the content of the mineral in consideration is higher than 150 mg per liter for calcium, 50 mg per liter for magnesium, 200 mg per liter for sodium, 200 mg per liter for sulfur, 1 mg per liter for fluorine, and 1 mg per liter for iron.

When two minerals are both present in high quantity, a combination classification is used—for example, "sodic-chlorine" water when the water in question contains a lot of chlorine and sodium; or "sulfurous-calcic" when sulfur and calcium are the predominant minerals. These designations are usually included with the labeling information on the bottles, which enables you to select the one best suited to your mineral needs.

When a specific deficiency needs to be remedied, choose one or more waters that are rich in the missing mineral and drink them daily over a four- to six-month period (see tables 7.1 through 7.7). If a particular deficiency is not the motive for taking the remedy, but you are trying to restore the overall mineral content of the body, you should drink a water rich in calcium, for example, the first month, perhaps a magnesium water the next month, and so on in any order you desire, so that the different kinds of waters and minerals follow one another in a series over time.

Water Used
Mineral and spring water exclusively.

Dosage
Drink when thirsty (dosage based on your normal habits) for a total of 2 liters a day.

Duration
Four to six months at the least when using commercially available waters. For mineral waters drunk at their source, especially when they have high mineral content, the duration of the remedy will be shorter. In such cases, you should obtain local guidance.

TABLE 7.1. WATERS RICH IN CALCIUM
(DAILY CALCIUM REQUIREMENT: 800 MG)

Name	mg/liter	Region of Origin
UNITED STATES		
Original Fountain of Youth Mineral Water	512	Florida
Manitou Mineral Water	290	Colorado
Colfax	180	Iowa
CANADA		
Abenakis	542	Quebec
IRELAND		
Roscommon	209	Roscommon
FRANCE		
Hépar	555	Lorraine
Contrex	467	Lorraine
Châteldon	420	Auvergne
Amélie la Reine	390	Rhône-Alps
Rozana	360	Auvergne

Name	Calcium mg/liter	Region of Origin
FRANCE (CONTINUED)		
Le Boulou	320	Languedoc-Roussillon
Oriol	307	Rhône-Alps
Wattwiller	288	Alsace
Salvetat	253	Languedoc-Roussillon
Quézac	252	Languedoc-Roussillon
Amanda	243	Nord-Pas-de-Calais
Orée du Bois	234	Nord-Pas-de-Calais
Vauban	230	Nord-Pas-de-Calais
Vittel	202	Lorraine
Badoit	200	Rhône-Alps
Sainte Marguerite	194	Auvergne
Vernière	190	Languedoc-Roussillon
Saint Alban	186	Rhône-Alps
Saint Amand	176	Nord-Pas-de-Calais
Arvie	170	Auvergne
Châteauneuf	162	Auvergne
SWITZERLAND		
San Bernardino	663	Calanca Valley
Alpenrose	569	Adelboden
Eptinger	555	Basel
Œybad-Quelle	532	Adelboden
Adello	505	Adelboden
Valser	436	Vals, Graubünden
Aproz	365	Valais
Mbudget	310	Aven
Lostorfer	279	Solothurn Canton
Passugger	211	Chur
Rhäzünser	210	Rhäzün
ITALY		
Fonte del Faro	1134	Tuscany
Acqua Arve	694	Parma
Pergoli di Tabiano	680	Pergoli
Acqua Regina	657	Tuscany
Acqua Fucoli	615	Tuscany

Name	Calcium mg/liter	Region of Origin
ITALY (CONTINUED)		
Bad Moos	560	Bozen
Fonti di Crodo	526	Piedmont
Piersanti	457	Livorno (Leghorn)
Acqua Tettucio	393	Pistoia
Telese	387	Benevento
Ferrarelle	362	Riardo
Vasciano	350	Perugia
Lavaredo	320	Merano
San Paolo	306	Rome
Acqua della Madonna	304	Naples
Fonte Santagata	270	Campania
San Silvestro	288	Brescia
Cinciano	283	Cinciano
Toka	248.5	Cavanna
Attiva	248	Tuscany
San Pellegrino	208	San Pellegrino Terme
GERMANY		
Bad Mergentheimer Albertquelle	794	Baden-Württemburg
Bad Mergentheimer Karlsquelle	750	Baden-Württemburg
Quellq Pur	625	Rottenburg Obernau
Teusser Medium	585	Teusserbad
Aqua Römer	572	Baden-Württemburg
Ensinger Mineralwasser	528	Baden-Württemburg
Alwa	485	Baden-Württemburg
Inesquelle	469	Löhne
Maxbrunnen Heilwasser	448	unavailable
Fortuna Quelle	380	Eichenzell
Fuldtaler	362	Malsfield
Extaler	350	Rinteln
Gerolsteiner Sprudel	347	Gerolstein
Bad Wildenger Helenenquelle	340	Hesse
Göppinger	313	Bavaria
Remstaler	300	Bavaria
Vulkania Heilwasser	277	Rhineland-Palatinate
Nürburgquelle	232	Rhineland-Palatinate

Name	Calcium mg/liter	Region of Origin
GERMANY (CONTINUED)		
Rosbacher Ur-Quelle	224	Rosbach vor der Höhe
Falkenbergquelle	218	Löhne
Merkur Classic	208	Hecklingen
Spreequell	208	Berlin
AUSTRIA		
Aubad Quelle	431	Tirol
Long Life	263	Stadtquelle Bad Radkersburg
Sound of Alps	244	Tirol
Juvina	240	Deutschkreuzbad
CZECH REPUBLIC		
Rudolph Quelle	276.7	Marienbad
Vincentka	245	Luhacovice
Saratica	219.7	Moravsky Beroun
SLOVAK REPUBLIC		
Sulinko	271.6	Presov
Lubovnianka	213	Lubovnianske Kupele
SPAIN		
Aguas de Manzanera	672	Teruel
Agua de Carabaña	505	Carabaña
Aquas Verdes	208	Fuerteventura

TABLE 7.2. WATERS RICH IN MAGNESIUM
(DAILY MAGNESIUM REQUIREMENT: 500–800 MG)

Name	mg/liter	Region of Origin
UNITED STATES		
Original Fountain of Youth Mineral Water	609	Florida
Noah's California Spring Water	110	San Antonio Valley
Adobe Springs	110	California
Colfax	91	Iowa
Deep Rock	60	Colorado

Name	Magnesium mg/liter	Region of Origin
CANADA		
Abenakis	320	Quebec
FRANCE		
Rozana	159	Auvergne
Sainte Marguerite	130	Auvergne
Le Boulou	126	Languedoc-Roussillon
Parot	94	Rhône-Alps
Arvie	92	Auvergne
Saint Diéry	90	Auvergne
Contrex	84	Lorraine
Amanda	77	Nord-Pas-de-Calais
Vernière	72	Languedoc-Roussillon
Orée du Bois	70	Nord-Pas-de-Calais
Reine des Basaltes	70	Rhône-Alps
Arcens	66	Rhône-Alps
Vauban	66	Nord-Pas-de-Calais
Saint Alban	63	Rhône-Alps
Nessel	52	Alsace
Châteldon	51	Auvergne
BELGIUM		
Léberg	47	Roosdal
SWITZERLAND		
Eptinger	127	Basel
San Bernardino	81	Calanca Valley
Lostorfer	78	Solothurn Canton
Mbudget	70	Aven
Aproz	67	Valais
Valser	54	Vals, Graubünden
Cristalp Saxon	40	Saxon
ITALY		
Attiva	578	Tuscany
San Lorenzo	315	Calabria
Acquarossa	151	Sicily
Vesuvio	143	Naples

Name	Magnesium mg/liter	Region of Origin
ITALY (CONTINUED)		
Acqua Arve	124	Parma
Acqua Regina	119	Tuscany
Piersanti	117	Livorno (Leghorn)
Ciappazzi	107	Messina
San Marco	91	Lazio
Acqua Fucoli	89	Tuscany
San Silvestro	80	Brescia
San Paolo	77	Roma
Telese	73	Benevento
Lavaredo	72	Merano
Donata	71.9	Tuscany
Santa Lucia	66	Sassari
Acqua Tettucio	64.4	Pistoia
Ausonia	63.6	Piedmont
Acqua della Madonna	62	Naples
Bad Moos	59	Bozen
Collalli	58	Tuscany
Vasciano	58	Perugia
Sant 'Andrea	56	Parma
San Pellegrino	55.9	San Pellegrino Terme
Pergoli di Tabiano	54	Pergoli
Ambra	52	Messina
Toka	50.6	Cavanna
SPAIN		
Agua de Carabaña	552	Carabaña
Aquas Verdes	256	Fuerteventura
Font del Pi	70.5	Alicante
Marmolejo	58	Jaén
Alhama	51	Almeria
Aqua de Sierra	51	Zaragoza
Font Sol	51	Valencia
CZECH REPUBLIC		
Saratica	943.8	Moravsky Beroun
Aqua Antonia	236	Marienbad

Name	Magnesium mg/liter	Region of Origin
CZECH REPUBLIC (CONTINUED)		
Magnesia	236	Carlsbad
Rudolph Quelle	136	Marienbad
Mostini	107	Horni Mostenice
SLOVAK REPUBLIC		
Sulinko	344.3	Presov
Lubovnianka	204.6	Lubovnianske Kupele
AUSTRIA		
Long Life	206	Stadtquelle Bad Radkersburg
Gleichenberger Johannisbrunnen	108	Steiermark
Römerquelle	65.6	Edelstal
Juvina	51	Deutschkreuzbad
GERMANY		
Kissinger Bitterwasser Heilwasser	4196	Bavaria
Bad Mergentheimer Albertquelle	783	Baden-Württemburg
Vulkania Heilwasser	380	Rhineland-Palatinate
Bad Mergentheimer Karlsquelle	376	Baden-Württemburg
Nürburgquelle	337	Rhineland-Palatinate
Dresier Sprudel	241	Rhineland-Palatinate
Bad Wildenger Helenenquelle	239	Hesse
Heppinger Extra	196	Ahrweiler
Maxbrunnen Heilwasser	149.6	unavailable
Apollinaris	130	Bad Neuenahr-Ahrweiler
Tonissteiner	130	Pönterquelle
Dunaris Heilwasser	126.6	Daun Rhineland-Palatinate
Ensinger Mineralwasser	124	Baden-Württemburg
Bad Driburger Bitterwasser	117	Eggegbirge
Reginaris	110	Mendig
Rosbacher Ur-Quelle	109	Rosbach vor der Höhe
Fuldtaler	108	Malsfield
Gerolsteiner Sprudel	108	Gerolstein
Adelheidquelle	102	Baden-Württemburg
Quellq Pur	87.5	Rottenburg Obernau

Name	Magnesium mg/liter	Region of Origin
GERMANY (CONTINUED)		
Teusser Medium	82	Teusserbad
Merkur Classic	80.5	Hecklingen
Adonis Heilwasser	80	Rhineland-Palatinate
Remstaler	70	Bavaria
Augusta Victoria	68	Hesse
Alwa	65.6	Baden-Württemburg
Göppinger	65	Bavaria
Inesquelle	62	Löhne
Falkenbergquelle	59	Löhne
Extaler	57	Rinteln
AUSTRALIA		
Boon Spa	50	Sailor Falls

TABLE 7.3. WATERS RICH IN SILICA

Name	mg/liter	Region of Origin
UNITED STATES		
Calistoga Mineral Water	145	California
Trinity Springs	74.6	Idaho
Calistoga Mountain Spring Water	55	California
Pagosa Springs	54	Colorado
Arrowhead	30.6	California (southern)
Palomar Mountain Spring Water	26.9	California (southern)
Parley's Canyon	14	Utah
CANADA		
Labrador	15	Labrador
Yukon Spring	9.9	Yukon
Naya (Mirabel)	7	Quebec
Malvern	10	English Midlands
Hydr8	8	Wales
Brecon Carreg	5.1	Wales

Name	Silica mg/liter	Region of Origin
IRELAND		
Fior Uisce	16.1	County Mayo
FRANCE		
Arvie	77	Auvergne
Salvetat	72	Languedoc-Roussillon
Ventadour	46	Rhône-Alps
Fontaine de Jouvence-Sail	39	Rhône-Alps
Puits St. Georges	38	Rhône-Alps
Chambon	36	Central France
Badoit	35	Rhône-Alps
BELGIUM		
Fertilia	28	Roosdaal
Spontin	19	Spontin
Spa Marie Henriette	15	Liège Province
Spa Barisart	10	Liège Province
SWITZERLAND		
Rhäzünser	50	Rhäzün
Knutwiler	17	Bad Knutwil
SPAIN		
Pinalito	135	Tenerife
Firgas	113	Grand Canary
Malavella	77.2	Girona
Vichy Catalan	76.8	Girona
Fonte Nova	61.8	Galicia
Aguas de Souzas	61	Verin
Fonte Celta	33	Galicia
Les Creus	23.6	Girona
Font Selva	22.5	Girona
Viladrau	22.5	Girona
Fonxestra	22	Galicia
Cabreiroa	18.2	Galicia
Font del Regàs	17.9	Girona
Agua de Mondariz	16.8	Pontevedra

Name	Silica mg/liter	Region of Origin
SPAIN (CONTINUED)		
Font D'or	14.2	Girona
Bezoya	11.2	Sierra de Guadarrama
Solan de Cabras	7.2	Cuenca
Fuente Sante	3.3	Asturias
PORTUGAL		
Carvelhelhos	41.9	Boticos
Frize	26.7	Vila Flor
São Cristóvão	17.9	Serra de Montemuro
Serrana	13.6	Cabril
Àgua do Fastio	13.5	Terras de Bouro
Alardo	12	Castelo Branco
ITALY		
San Petro	104	Rome
Giulia	102	Rome
Leggera	102	Monticchio Bagni
Ninfa	100	Basilicata
Appia	96.2	Appia
San Paolo	95	Rome
Ferrarelle	81	Riardo
Fontesana	76	Fontesana
Fonte Giulia	74	Rome
Acqua Arve	70	Parma
Fonte Santagata	63	Campania
Collalli	61	Tuscany
San Lorenzo	60	Calabria
San Marco	58	Lazio
Piersanti	55	Livorno (Leghorn)
Vesuvio	55	Naples
Pergoli di Tabiano	50	Pergoli
Attiva	49	Tuscany
Santa Lucia	45	Sassari
Ciappazzi	44	Messina
Fonte Lidia	42.5	Parma
Acqua della Madonna	37	Naples

Name	Silica mg/liter	Region of Origin
ITALY (CONTINUED)		
Ausonia	29	Piedmont
Donata	27	Tuscany
Montinverno	25	Parma
Mitterbad	22	Bozen
Luce	21.7	Cagliari
Vasciano	21.4	Perugia
Cinciano	20.4	Cinciano
Gerasia	20.4	Sicily
Fonte Meo	17.5	Rome
Vigezzo	16.7	Piedmont
Pic	10.7	Turin
Roccabianca	9.2	Sicily
San Pellegrino	9	San Pellegrino Terme
Dolomiti	7.3	Valli del Pasubia
Azzurina	7	Betulla
Misia	6.8	Perugia
Vaia	6.6	Brescia
Daggio	6.4	Lombardy
Santa Rita	6	Genoa
Ducale	5.4	Parma (Monte Zuccone)
GERMANY		
Dunaris Heilwasser	75	Daun Rhineland-Palatinate
König Otto-Sprudel	69.5	Wiesau
Tonissteiner	52	Pönterquelle
Gerolsteiner Sprudel	40.2	Gerolstein
Heppinger Extra	38	Ahrweiler
Bad Wildenger Helenenquelle	36.4	Hesse
Aquella	34.1	Bochum
Wittenseer Quelle	30.4	Berlin
Randegger Ottilien-Quelle	20	Baden-Württemburg
St. Leonhardsquelle	15	Rosenheim
Eiszeitquell	14.8	Baden-Württemburg
Staatl. Bad Brückenauer	14.74	Bavaria
Bad Mergentheimer Karlsquelle	12	Baden-Württemburg

Name	Silica mg/liter	Region of Origin
AUSTRIA		
Waldquelle	42.6	Kobersdorf
Gasteiner	13.4	Bad Gastein
CZECH REPUBLIC		
Mylynsky	73.7	Karlsbad
Aqua Antonia	71	Marienbad
Magnesia	71	Carlsbad
Bilinska Kyselka	52.1	Bilina
AUSTRALIA		
Mount Seaview Spring Water	53	New South Wales
Tasmanian Highland Spring Waters	40	Huon Valley
Boon Spa	21	Sailor Falls
Hartz Mineral Water	20	Huon Region
NEW ZEALAND		
Eternal Water	85	Bay of Plenty
SnoZone	18.8	Hihitahi
Waimak	18	South Island
Edge	18	South Island
New Zealand Crew	18	South Island
Virgin Kiwi	18	South Island

TABLE 7.4. WATERS RICH IN IRON

Name	mg/liter	Region of Origin
UNITED STATES		
Palomar Mountain Spring Water	0.7	California (southern)
Pagosa Springs	0.08	Colorado
UNITED KINGDOM		
Hadrian	0.02	Northumbria
Scotch Mist	0.02	Scotland
Blue Keld	0.007	East Yorkshire

Name	Iron mg/liter	Region of Origin
IRELAND		
Aveta Celtic Goddess of Healing Waters	39.4	Oyster Haven
ICELAND		
Thorspring	0.03	Reykjavik
Ice Blue	0.01	Thorlakshofn
FRANCE		
Hépar	10	Lorraine
ITALY		
Montinverno	815	Parma
Flitz	219.4	Bozen
Mitterbad	70	Bozen
SPAIN		
Malavella	0.39	Girona
Font D'or	0.1	Girona
Vichy Catalan	0.1	Girona
Font del Regàs	0.03	Girona
Aquas Verdes	0.05	Fuerteventura
GERMANY		
Bad Mergentheimer Albertquelle	9.73	Baden-Württemburg
Vulkania Heilwasser	9.5	Rhineland-Palatinate
Maxbrunnen Heilwasser	7.3	unavailable
Bad Wildenger Helenenquelle	5.4	Hesse
St. Leonhardsquelle	3.7	Rosenheim
Bad Mergentheimer Karlsquelle	2.6	Baden-Württemburg
Eiszeitquell	1.4	Baden-Würtemburg
Staatl. Bad Brückenauer	0.02	Bavaria
Heppinger Extra	0.02	Ahrweiler
Wernarzer Heilwasser	0.01	Bad Brücknau
Randegger Ottilien-Quelle	0.009	Baden-Würtemburg

Name	Iron mg/liter	Region of Origin
AUSTRIA		
Gleichenberger Johannisbrunnen	6.3	Steiermark
Long Life	2.6	Stadtquelle Bad Radkersburg
Triple A	0.02	Quelle Thalheim
Römerquelle	0.0047	Edelstal
Oxygiser	0.004	Tyrol
CZECH REPUBLIC		
Rudolph Quelle	12	Marienbad
Vincentka	7	Luhacovice
Mostini	2.45	Horni Mostenice
SLOVAK REPUBLIC		
Lubovnianka	0.3	Lubovnianske Kupele
Cigel Spring Water	0.091	Bardejov
POLAND		
DEA	0.3	Polczyn Zdroj
SWEDEN		
Malmburg Original Water	0.33	Ynasjö
AUSTRALIA		
Boon Spa	6.4	Sailor Falls
Emerald Forest	0.16	New South Wales
Tasmanian Highland Spring Waters	0.05	Huon Valley

TABLE 7.5. WATERS RICH IN MANGANESE

Name	mg/liter	Region of Origin
UNITED STATES		
Manitou Mineral Water	0.14	Colorado
Pagosa Springs	0.023	Colorado
CANADA		
Sahara Water	0.01	unavailable

Name	Manganese mg/liter	Region of Origin
ICELAND		
Ice Blue	0.01	Thorlakshofn
FRANCE		
Hépar	3.5	Lorraine
Reine des Basaltes	0.6	Rhône-Alps
Le Boulou	0.35	Languedoc-Roussillon
ITALY		
Flitz	10.65	Bozen
Mitterbad	1.57	Bozen
Fonte Giulia	0.5	Rome
SPAIN		
Aquas Verdes	0.02	Fuerteventura
Font D'or	0.02	Girona
Font del Regàs	0.02	Girona
Malavella	0.02	Girona
Vichy Catalan	0.02	Girona
GERMANY		
Maxbrunnen Heilwasser	0.96	unavailable
Bad Mergentheimer Albertquelle	0.95	Baden-Württemburg
Vulkania Heilwasser	0.72	Rhineland-Palatinate
Gerolsteiner Sprudel	0.4	Rhineland-Palatinate
Bad Wildenger Helenenquelle	0.36	Hesse
Wernarzer Heilwasser	0.31	Bad Brücknau
Randegger Ottilien-Quelle	0.19	Baden-Württemburg
St. Leonhardsquelle	0.18	Rosenheim
Eiszeitquell	0.15	Baden-Württemburg
Adonis Heilwasser	0.12	Rhineland-Palatinate
Bad Mergentheimer Karlsquelle	0.11	Baden-Württemburg
Heppinger Extra	0.056	Ahrweiler
Staatl. Bad Brückenauer	0.02	Bavaria
Wittenseer Quelle	0.005	Berlin
AUSTRIA		
Alps	10.4	Frankenmarkt, Salzkammergut

Name	Manganese mg/liter	Region of Origin
AUSTRIA (CONTINUED)		
Triple A	0.02	Quelle Thalheim
Oxygiser	0.004	Tyrol
Römerquelle	0.0026	Edelstal
CZECH REPUBLIC		
Aqua Maria	1.36	Marienbad
Vincentka	0.6	Luhacovice
Rudolph Quelle	0.548	Marienbad
SLOVAK REPUBLIC		
Lubovnianka	0.35	Lubovnianske Kupele
Cigel Spring Water	0.013	Bardejov
POLAND		
DEA	0.09	Polczyn Zdroj
SWEDEN		
Malmburg Original Water	0.03	Ynasjö
AUSTRALIA		
Boon Spa	0.14	Sailor Falls
Winfred Springs	0.03	Rylstone
Tasmanian Highland Spring Waters	0.01	Tasmania

TABLE 7.6. WATERS RICH IN LITHIUM

Name	mg/liter	Region of Origin
UNITED STATES		
Arrowhead	7.8	California (southern)
Pagosa Springs	2.9	Colorado
Manitou Mineral Water	0.24	Colorado
Famous Crazy Mineral Water	0.009	Texas
IRELAND		
Fior Uisce	0.242	County Mayo

Name	Lithium mg/liter	Region of Origin
FRANCE		
Hépar	70	Lorraine
Quézac	1.5	Languedoc-Roussillon
SPAIN		
Fonte Nova	2.9	Galicia
Malavella	1.31	Girona
Vichy Catalan	1.31	Girona
Aquas Verdes	0.01	Fuerteventura
GERMANY		
Bad Mergentheimer Albertquelle	13.3	Baden-Württemburg
Bad Mergentheimer Karlsquelle	5.8	Baden-Württemburg
Heppinger Extra	1.1	Ahrweiler
Bad Wildenger Helenenquelle	0.71	Hesse
Staatl. Bad Brückenauer	0.05	Bavaria
Eiszeitquell	0.016	Baden-Würtemburg
Randegger Ottilien-Quelle	0.015	Baden-Würtemburg
AUSTRIA		
Adonis Heilwasser	290	Rhineland-Palatinate
Römerquelle	0.0025	Edelstal
CZECH REPUBLIC		
Aqua Maria	34.5	Marienbad
Vincentka	27.5	Luhacovice
Bilinska Kyselka	3.67	Bilina
Mylynsky	2.75	Karlsbad
Saratica	1.1	Moravsky Beroun
SLOVAK REPUBLIC		
Sulinko	3.55	Presov
Lubovnianka	0.16	Lubovnianske Kupele
Cigel Spring Water	0.094	Bardejov

TABLE 7.7. WATERS RICH IN ZINC

Name	mg/liter	Region of Origin
UNITED STATES		
Famous Crazy Mineral Water	0.972	Texas
Manitou Mineral Water	0.21	Colorado
Pagosa Springs	0.01	Colorado
Mountain Valley Spring	0.01	Arkansas
CANADA		
Naya (Revelstoke)	0.05	British Columbia
Naya (Saint André Est)	0.05	Quebec
Naya (Mirabel)	0.05	Quebec
Empress Springs	0.034	Saanich Peninsula
Sahara Water	0.02	unavailable
UNITED KINGDOM		
Kingshill Forest Glade	0.1	Scotland (Lanarkshire)
FRANCE		
Hépar	3	Lorraine
ITALY		
Flitz	1.575	Bozen
GERMANY		
Adonis Heilwasser	20	Rhineland-Palatinate
Vulkania Heilwasser	0.015	Rhineland-Palatinate
St. Leonhardsquelle	0.01	Rosehheim
AUSTRIA		
Alps	25.4	Frankenmarkt, Salzkammergut
Gasteiner	0.05	Bad Gastein
Römerquelle	0.015	Edelstal
Oxygiser	0.009	Tyrol
SLOVAK REPUBLIC		
Cigel Spring Water	0.053	Bardejov
Lubovnianka	0.020	Lubovnianske Kupele

Name	Zinc mg/liter	Region of Origin
AUSTRALIA		
Wattle Springs	0.05	Sutton Forest
Tasmanian Highland Spring Waters	0.01	Huon Valley
Winfred Springs	0.01	Rylstone

HYDRATION AND DEACIDIFICATION REMEDY

This remedy aims simultaneously to hydrate the tissues and deacidify the internal cellular environment of the body. Normally, an alkaline–acid imbalance with acid predominating can be corrected by following an alkaline diet.* Drinking alkaline water acts in the same fashion.

Method
Select the 2 liters of water you drink a day from mineral waters and springs rich in alkaline minerals, meaning waters whose pH is higher than 7.

How It Works
The alkaline minerals contained in the water neutralize the excess acids responsible for acidifying the body's internal cellular environment. Furthermore, the neutral salts created as a result (one alkaline and one acid equal one neutral salt) are easily evacuated by the kidneys and sudoriferous glands, thanks to the substantial volume of water being ingested.

Water Used
An alkaline mineral water or water from an alkaline spring (see table 7.8). Or tap water or distilled water whose pH has

---

*For further information, and to determine whether you have an acid–alkaline imbalance, see my book *The Acid–Alkaline Diet for Optimum Health*.

been increased to 9 or 9.5 with the help of an alkalizing agent, also called pH drops. (See phion Nutrition in the resources section.)

Dosage
Drink 2 liters (one half-gallon) a day when thirsty (based on your normal drinking habits).

Duration
Four to six months at minimum. For people who are extremely acidified, an entire year.

TABLE 7.8. ALKALINE MINERAL WATERS

Name	pH	Region of Origin
UNITED STATES		
Trinity Springs	9.7	Idaho
Rain	9	Utah
Alaska Chill	8.85	Alaska
Adobe Springs	8.4	California
Noah's California Spring Water	8.3	San Antonio Valley
Deer Park	8.05	Maryland
Loon Country	8.05	Maine
Crystal Geyser Natural Spring Water	7.9	California
EartH2O	7.9	Oregon
Mountain Valley Spring Water	7.8	Arkansas
Seven Creeks Spring Water	7.78	Ohio
Calistoga Mineral Water	7.7	California
English Mountain	7.7	Tennessee
Hawaiian Springs Natural Water	7.7	Hawaii
Zephyrhills	7.7	Florida

Name	pH	Region of Origin
UNITED STATES (CONTINUED)		
Giant Springs	7.6	Montana
Hinkley & Schmitt	7.6	California (southern)
Diamond Natural Spring Water	7.58	Arkansas (Hot Springs)
Fountainhead	7.5	South Carolina
Calistoga Mountain Spring Water	7.46	California
Colfax	7.4	Iowa
Palomar Mountain Spring Water	7.4	California (southern)
Keeper Springs	7.39	Vermont
Cobb Mountain	7.3	California (northern)
Sparkletts	7.3	California
Mount Olympus	7.24	Utah
Vermont Pure	7.2	Vermont
Colorado Crystal	7	Colorado
Manitou Mineral Water	7	Colorado
CANADA		
Empress Springs	8.32	Saanich Peninsula
Cedar Springs	8.1	Ontario (Oro Mountain)
Mountain Lite	8.1	Alberta
Naya (Revelstoke)	7.8	British Columbia
Naya (Saint André Est)	7.8	Quebec
Monashee	7.57	British Columbia
Kootenay Spring	7.5	British Columbia
Naya (Mirabel)	7.5	Quebec
Rocky Mountain Spring	7.4	Alberta
Whistler Water Pure Glacial Spring	7.3	British Columbia
Yukon Spring	7.29	Yukon
Canoe Springs	7.16	Ontario
Aquafina	7	Quebec
MEXICO		
Agua Manatial	8	Acapulco
Santa Maria	7.2	Lomas de Chapultepec

Name	pH	Region of Origin
COSTA RICA		
Cristal	7.7	Heredia
UNITED KINGDOM		
Abbey Well	7.9	Northumbria
Brecon Carreg	7.8	Wales
Cotswold Spring	7.8	Bristol
Highland Spring	7.8	Scotland
Shepley Spring	7.8	West Yorkshire
Springhill	7.8	North Yorkshire
Celtic Spring	7.7	Longtown
Blue Keld	7.6	East Yorkshire
Galloway	7.6	Scotland
Buxton	7.4	Derbyshire
Glendale Spring	7.4	Scotland (Perthshire)
Wildboarclough	7.3	Cheshire
Findlay	7.2	Scotland
Hadrian	7.2	Northumbria
Glen Orrin	7	Scotland
IRELAND		
Fior Uisce	7.8	County Mayo
Tipperary	7.7	Barrisoleigh
Aveta Celtic Goddess of Healing Waters	7.5	Oyster Haven
Ballygowan	7.2	County Kerry (Newcastle West)
Galway	7.2	Galway
Nash's	7.2	County Kerry (Newcastle West)
Silver Stone	7.2	Donegal
ICELAND		
Ice Blue	7.9	Thorlakshofn
FRANCE		
Montclar	8	Provence-Alps-Côte d'Azur
Luchon	8	Midi-Pyrenees

Name	pH	Region of Origin
FRANCE (CONTINUED)		
Chantereine	7.9	Ile-de-France
Pyrénées	7.9	Midi-Pyrenees
Cristaline-Neyrolles	7.8	Rhône-Alps
Cristaline-Sainte Cécile	7.6	Provence-Alps-Côte d'Azur
Fontan	7.6	Provence-Alps-Côte d'Azur
Laurier	7.6	Ile-de-France
Ogeu	7.6	Aquitaine
Roche des Écrins	7.6	Provence-Alps-Côte d'Azur
Sainte-Anne des Abatilles	7.5	Aquitaine
Amanda	7.5	Nord-Pas-de-Calais
Cristaline-Grand Bois	7.5	Champagne-Ardennes
Cristaline-La Bondoire St. Hippolyte	7.5	Central France
Cristaline-Saint Médard	7.5	Aquitaine
Fontaine de Jouvence-Sail	7.5	Rhône-Alps
Wattwiller	7.5	Alsace
Alet	7.4	Languedoc-Roussillon
Bompart	7.4	Poitou-Charentes
Cristaline-St. Cyr La Source	7.4	Central France
La Fiée des Lois	7.4	Poitou-Charentes
Mont-Dore	7.4	Auvergne
Roxane	7.4	Loire Valley
Saint Léger	7.4	Nord-Pas-de-Calais
Thonon	7.4	Rhône-Alps
Aix	7.3	Rhône-Alps
Chambon	7.3	Central France
Contrex	7.3	Lorraine
Elvina-Dax	7.3	Aquitaine
Evian	7.2	Rhône-Alps
Vittel	7.2	Lorraine
Orée du Bois	7.1	Nord-Pas-de-Calais
Pierval	7.1	Normandy
Saint Christophe	7.1	Aquitaine
Vauban	7.1	Nord-Pas-de-Calais

Name	pH	Region of Origin
FRANCE (CONTINUED)		
Hépar	7	Lorraine
Saint Amand	7	Nord-Pas-de-Calais
Vals Saint Lambert	7	Ile-de-France
Ventadour	7	Rhône-Alps
Volvic	7	Auvergne
BELGIUM		
Valvert	7.7	Ardennes
Val d'Aisne	7.5	Aisne Valley
Spontin	7.3	Spontin
Chaufontaine	7	Ardennes
Villers	7	Villers le Gambon
SWITZERLAND		
Eden Dorénaz	7.8	Valais (Wallis Canton)
Knutwiler	7.7	Bad Knutwil
Nendaz	7.6	Valais
Henniez Bleu	7.5	Vaud Canton
GERMANY		
St. Leonhardsquelle	7.68	Rosenheim
Wittenseer Quelle	7.3	Berlin
Randegger Ottilien-Quelle	7.26	Baden-Würtemburg
Eiszeitquell	7.04	Baden-Würtemburg
AUSTRIA		
Alps	7.85	Frankenmarkt, Salzkammergut
Siberquelle	7.6	Brixlegg
Triple A	7.5	Quelle Thalheim
Oxygiser	7.52	Tyrol
ITALY		
Fonte Lidia	9.3	Parma
Valmora	8.4	Aburu
Ducale	8.3	Parma (Monte Zuccone)
Pradis	8.2	Friuli-Venezia Giulia
Vaia	8.2	Brescia

Name	pH	Region of Origin
ITALY (CONTINUED)		
Dolomiti	8.18	Valli del Pasubia
Attiva	8.1	Tuscany
Azzurina	8.1	Betulla
Vigezzo	8.1	Piedmont
Coralba	8	Ischia
Pic	8	Turin
Santa Rita	8	Genoa
Monte Bianco	7.9	Aosta
Monviso	7.9	Turin
Motette	7.9	Perugia
Pineta	7.9	Lombardy
Fonte Laura	7.8	Como
Misia	7.72	Perugia
San Pellegrino	7.7	San Pellegrino Terme
Luce	7.66	Cagliari
Roccabianca	7.65	Sicily
Balda	7.6	Veneto
Fonti di Crodo	7.6	Piedmont
Sant Andrea	7.6	Parma
Gerasia	7.42	Sicily
Daggio	7.4	Lombardy
Lavaredo	7.4	Merano
Ciappazzi	7.2	Messina
Collalli	7.2	Tuscany
Montinverno	7.2	Parma
Fonte Meo	7.08	Rome
SPAIN		
Font del Regàs	8.08	Girona
Font D'or	8.2	Girona
Viladrau	7.4	Girona
Les Creus	7	Girona
Font Vella	7.62	Girona
Sousas	7.52	Galicia
Aquas Verdes	7.4	Fuerteventura
Solan de Cabras	7.4	Cuenca
Fuente Sante	7	Asturias

Name	pH	Region of Origin
PORTUGAL		
Monchique	9.5	Pancados
Carvelhelhos	7.82	Boticos
Castelo de Vide	7.4	Alentejo
Pizões	7.2	Moura
SLOVAK REPUBLIC		
Cigel Spring Water	7.98	Bardejov
Ludovicus	7.82	Bardejov
SWEDEN		
Malmburg Original Water	7.9	Ynasjö
AUSTRALIA		
Mount Seaview Spring Water	8.5	New South Wales
Gigis Water	7.62	Victoria
Entee	7.5	Northern Territory (Darwin)
Boon Spa	7.3	Sailor Falls
Wattle Springs	7.1	Sutton Forest
NEW ZEALAND		
SnoZone	8	Hihitahi
Waimak	7.9	South Island
Edge	7.9	South Island
New Zealand Crew	7.9	South Island
Virgin Kiwi	7.9	South Island
Eternal Water	7	Bay of Plenty

HYDRATION AND SPORTS

Athletes must make sure their bodies are well hydrated before, during, and after engaging in their chosen sport to give themselves the maximum compensation for the water they will inevitably lose (in the form of sweat) during strenuous physical exercise. The problem for athletes (and physical laborers) is that the more liquid they lose, the less effective they become. This does not pose much of a dilemma for short-term efforts (less than an hour), but it becomes a fundamental problem during prolonged efforts.

Method

There are four specific times that should be taken into consideration.

Before the activity. Over the course of a year, you should regularly use Rehydration Remedy #1 or #2 (see pages 108–11) to ensure that the tissues contain the maximum amount of water physiologically possible. This way you will not go into your sports activities already suffering from a water deficiency.

Directly before the activity. It is a good idea to supply your body with a certain quantity of water just prior to engaging in a demanding physical effort. This enables the body to compensate rapidly for the initial fluid loss without having to make deductions from the tissues, and thus from the muscles.

This quantity should not be too large, however. The intestines' capacity to absorb water is limited to about 20 to 34 ounces (600 ml to 1 liter) an hour. Any more than that will sit stagnant and upset your stomach. An overly large volume of water can also cause hyperhydration of the tissues, requiring you to urinate during your sports activity, which is obviously not desirable. The right amount is about 18 ounces (5 deciliters) of water drunk around a half hour to an hour before the activity begins; do not drink anything for the final half hour.

During the activity. It is not always easy to drink during an athletic activity but, with a liter or more of sweat lost in an hour, it is imperative to replenish some of this water. The most physiologically effective method is to drink a little at a time, but often—for example, 4 to 6 ounces (1 to 2 deciliters) every ten to fifteen minutes.

After the activity. There is always a hydric deficiency following any strenuous physical effort, because the elimination of water by the skin (1 to 3 liters an hour) is higher than the intestines' assimilating capacities. The length of time required for rehydration depends on how deeply the body has been dehydrated. It can take up to 3 liters in four hours at a rate of 3 to 7 ounces (1 to 2 deciliters) every fifteen minutes. The speed of assimilation does not depend at all on the state of dehydration the body is experiencing; it is a fixed amount.

Water Used

Mineral or spring water to make up for any mineral depletion; slightly sweetened water to combat sudden fatigue due to hypoglycemia; or slightly salted water (1 gram per liter) to encourage intestinal assimilation and make up for the loss of sodium caused by sweating—but this is only necessary when sweating has been intense.

Note

Only broad principles of hydration for athletes have been outlined here. For more details, there are books that address this subject in depth (see the bibliography).

HYDRATION AND BEAUTY

Although beauty is largely a matter of inner radiance, physical treatments can help keep us feeling and looking our best. Water remedies can be quite effective in maintaining the figure and skin in particular.

The figure. Weight gain from overeating can cause unflattering changes to the figure, but it can be fought with a water remedy. By drinking generous amounts of water (more than 2 liters, or a half-gallon a day), you can reduce the amount of food consumed and also eliminate false hunger pangs.

Furthermore, good hydration of the tissues encourages enzymatic activity and therefore the burning of fat deposits. (See pages 52–53.)

The skin. Water is an essential ingredient for skin regeneration. The skin of a 130-pound individual contains around 2 gallons of water, and the skin of a 160-pound individual contains almost 2.5 gallons of water. This water is retained by special molecules capable of holding in place a thousand times their weight in water. Dehydration is one of the principal factors in the aging of the skin and the loss of a fresh youthful appearance.

When the skin lacks water, it becomes dull, dry, and wrinkled and loses its elasticity, firmness, and color. Pimple outbreaks become more common because the sudoriferous and sebaceous glands eliminate toxins poorly and become congested.

Hydrating the skin properly by drinking enough prevents these assaults on the skin or banishes them if they are already occurring.

Water Used

Spring water or mineral water with low mineral content (total dissolved solids in quantities of less than 500 mg/liter; see table 5.2 on pages 72–81).

Dosage

To lose weight, drink 2.5 to 3.5 liters or more of water per day. The quantity should be based on your weight (more weight equals more water) and the amount you eat.

To maintain youthful skin, around 2.5 liters of water a day should be sufficient.

Duration

To be effective, these remedies should be followed for the long term.

Bibliography

Batmanghelidj, Fereydoon. *Your Body's Many Cries for Water.* 2nd edition. Vienna, Va.: Global Health Solutions, 1992.

Clark, Nancy. *Nancy Clark's Sports Nutrition Guidebook.* 3rd edition. Champaign, Ill.: Human Kinetics Publishers, 2003.

Garnier, Alain. *Alimentation et sport* [Diet and Sports]. Paris: Éditions Maloine, 1992.

Ingram, Colin. *The Drinking Water Book: How to Eliminate the Most Harmful Toxins from Your Water.* 2nd edition. Berkeley, Calif.: Celestial Arts, 2006.

Manteuffel-Szoege, Leon. "Réflexions sur la nature des functions mécaniques du coeur" [Thoughts on the Heart's Mechanical Functions]. *Minerva Cardioangiologica Europea,* VI, 1958.

Ryan, Monique. *Sports Nutrition for Endurance Athletes.* Boulder, Colo.: VeloPress, 2002.

Vasey, Christopher. *The Acid–Alkaline Diet for Optimum Health.* Rochester, Vt.: Healing Arts Press, 2003.

———. *The Whey Prescription.* Rochester, Vt.: Healing Arts Press, forthcoming 2006.

Resources

Mineral Waters of the World
www.mineralwaters.org

The world's leading water directory—includes waters listed by country with nutritional information, consumer ratings, and water facts.

BOTTLED WATER WHOLESALERS

The following companies sell bottled waters from around the world:

Aqua Maestro
1460 N.W. First Court • Boca Raton, FL 33423
561-392-3336, ext. 102
www.aquamaestro.com

The Bottled Water Store
P.O. Box 880375 • Boca Raton, FL 33488
888-225-6222
www.bottledwaterstore.com

SUPPLEMENTS
phion Nutrition
7741 E Gray Rd, Suite 9 • Scottsdale AZ 85260
888-744-8589
www.ph-ion.com

phion Nutrition is a manufacturer and distributor of products geared toward augmenting healthy body chemistry. Contact phion Nutrition or go to their Web site for further information about, or to order, the Alkalive pH booster for structured alkaline water.

Index

Page numbers in italics refer to figures and tables.